Abstinence

2nd Edition

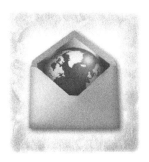

Members of
Overeaters Anonymous
Share Their Experience, Strength,
and Hope

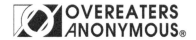

ISBN 978-1-889681-38-2

Library of Congress Control No: 2012916611

Overeaters Anonymous®, Inc.

World Service Office

6075 Zenith Court

Rio Rancho, NM 87144

Mail Address: P.O. Box 44727

Rio Rancho, NM 87174-4727

(505) 891-2664

www.oa.org

OA Board-Approved

©1994, 2013 by Overeaters Anonymous, Inc.

First Edition 1994.

Second Edition 2013.

All rights reserved.

Second printing 2021.

Printed in the United States of America

PREFACE

This book is a collection of stories and essays on the topic of abstinence. All were written by members of the Overeaters Anonymous Fellowship and were published in *Lifeline*, OA's international magazine of recovery. The opinions expressed are those of the individual writers and do not represent OA as a whole. Their words are not intended to give a definitive or ideological answer to our questions about abstinence; rather, they represent to us many different examples of experience, strength, and hope.

Whether you are a longtimer with many years of abstinence, a member struggling with recovery or relapse, or a newcomer to whom the subject of abstinence may still be a mystery, may you find encouragement, help, and direction within these pages.

**Overeaters Anonymous Policy on Abstinence and Recovery
(adopted in 1988; amended in 2002, 2009, 2011, and 2019)**

The WSBC 2019 accepts the following definitions:
1. Abstinence: The act of refraining from compulsive eating and compulsive food behaviors while working towards or maintaining a healthy body weight.
2. Recovery: Removal of the need to engage in compulsive eating behaviors.
Spiritual, emotional, and physical recovery is achieved through working and living the Overeaters Anonymous Twelve Step program.

CONTENTS

CHAPTER ONE
The Meaning of Abstinence

1962–Abstinence Enters OA 2	A State of Grace 10
The Year of Abstinence Awareness 5	It's Simple and It Works 11
	Freedom of Choice 12
Positive Result 6	Inseparable Solution 15
Reaching for the Promises 7	Perplexed About Abstinence? .. 17
Quiet Reaffirmation 8	Say Yes to Abstinence 19

CHAPTER TWO
Practical Ways to Achieve Abstinence

Food Corral 22	Crystal Clear 35
Building the Foundation 23	Time-Tested Recovery 36
Step One Situation 25	It's All in the Steps 38
What Is a Healthy Weight? 26	Formula for Living 41
In the Field 27	Aussie "How-To" 42
Relapse Prevention 28	Finally, Abstinence 44
Condition Check 30	Abstinent in Pastry Hell 45
Plugging the Dam 32	Gift of Abstinence 46
Travel Insurance 34	You Can Too 47

CHAPTER THREE
The Search for Abstinence

Perfect Shift 50	Taking My Medicine 61
A Misguided Goal 51	The Reprieve. 63
Getting Back Up 52	It Works if You Work It. 64
Coming Clean 52	Worthwhile Struggle 66
No More Traffic Cop 54	It's a Personal Choice 68
The Moment it Clicked. 55	Crucial Step 68
Living in the Solution 57	Abstinent and Smoke-Free. 70
Trust to the Test. 58	Footwork of Abstinence 72
Back in the Game 60	

CHAPTER FOUR
Abstinence Is a Priority

Stick Around 74	The Abstinence Advantage. 81
No Matter What 75	Abstinence–
Bye-Bye, Seconds 76	It's Not a Numbers Game . . . 83
Taking Action. 77	Handle With Care 84
A Pivotal Decision. 79	Clear Intention. 86

CHAPTER FIVE
Abstinence and The Tools

A Choice I Make 88	Serenity in A Suitcase 94
Abstinent Sponsors 89	Taming the Bear 95
Fit Food Around Life 91	Sharing Thanks 96
Hidden Part 92	Following Directions. 97
The Pen Is Mightier Than	My Maintenance Checklist. 98
the Relapse 93	Simple Plan. 100

CHAPTER SIX
Abstinent Living

Keeping Food Where It Belongs 102
I'm Okay 103
What Is "Normal"? 104
So Grateful 105
If You Work It 106
Gains and Losses 107
This Girl's Tale 108
Finding the Miracle 110
Right Now 112
An Abstinent Vacation 113
Sweet Surrender 114
Moving Ahead 116
Recovery Roster 118
Present for Life 119
Finding the Balance 120
Feeling Full 122
Party Plan 123
The Tempest 124
The Ghost of Christmas Past .. 125
An OA Lexicon 127
Island Oasis 128
Promising Steps 131
New Way of Living 133
Livin' It Up! 134
You Can Take It With You 135
Abstinence Has No Boundaries 136
Flying High With OA 137
No Games With the Food 138
Maintaining Long-Term Abstinence 140
Joint Effort 142
New Day, New Life 143
Thanksgiving Anniversary 145
Pregnancy and Recovery 146

CHAPTER SEVEN
How Abstinence Changes with Time and Experience

Still Works 150
Most Important Thing 151
Blessed Event 152
Opening Windows 153
Perfection Not Required 154
Relapse Happens 155
Progress Report 157
An Amazing, Abstinent Life .. 159
The Relief of Honesty 161
No Person, Place, or Thing 162

CHAPTER EIGHT
What Abstinence Has Taught Me

Great Equalizer 166	A Bouquet For Abstinence.... 172
Life After Loss 167	Young and Abstinent......... 174
Thursday Night Friends 168	Standouts 175
Plugged Into Recovery 170	
The Importance of Being Honest 171	

The Twelve Steps of Overeaters Anonymous.................. 178

The Twelve Traditions of Overeaters Anonymous 179

CHAPTER ONE

The Meaning of Abstinence

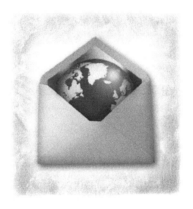

Rozanne S., OA's founder, explains how the concept of abstinence emerged

1962—Abstinence Enters OA

Eager for information about our early years, members frequently ask me: "How did the idea of abstinence come into OA? Was it always the way it is today? How did it start?"

Looking back, the years from 1960-1962 were exciting for us. We were so impulsive, so eager to see our tiny Fellowship grow and establish a firm foundation. By 1962 we were united about the wording of our Twelve Steps and Twelve Traditions. In other areas, however, we all had different ideas on how to achieve our common goals.

> *Together we can climb those Twelve Steps to recovery, abstaining from compulsive overeating one day at a time!*

Consider food intake, for example. Before 1960 most of us had grown up counting calories. We had been taught that as long as we kept within our calorie count, we could eat all the barely caloric foods we wanted between meals.

Our problem was that while many of us had lost weight, even more were nibbling their way back to obesity. Others were sticking with their diets but crunching all day on the low-cal foods. Many just stayed fat, insisting they were only eating allowable foods between meals. Something crucial was missing. What was it? The Twelve Steps worked for our Alcoholics Anonymous (AA) friends; what were we doing wrong?

During those years I was going to AA meetings every week. Although I'm not an alcoholic, my understanding of the Steps and Traditions was so limited I believed I could learn more by attending AA.

In early 1962, one powerful AA meeting changed my way of thinking about eating. All through that meeting the speakers emphasized "abstinence" from alcohol. During the two years I'd had contact with AA, I had never heard sobriety referred to in that manner. It was a revelation!

Sitting in the back of that meeting, I thought to myself: "That's what's wrong with all of us in OA. We're not abstaining from food at any time of the day. We have to close our mouths from the end of one meal to the beginning of the next. Sometime during the day, we must 'abstain' from eating; otherwise we're feeding our compulsion."

Excitedly I brought my new approach back to OA. Some thought it was a breakthrough; others scoffed.

By spring of 1962 we counted nineteen OA groups, most of them in California. The OA office was in my little dining room, and I was the unofficial, unpaid national secretary. We had already had our first informal meeting of the Los Angeles area groups; now we agreed it was time to have a real conference of all OA groups.

Therefore, in May 1962 I sent out an *Overeaters Anonymous Bulletin* (forerunner of today's *Lifeline*) to all OA groups. It introduced secretaries and group starters to one another and mentioned the proposed Conference.

Then on page three of that first *Bulletin* came the announcement that would both unify and upset us for decades:

"Out of our regular visits to AA meetings and talks with our friends in Alcoholics Anonymous, we here in the Los Angeles area have discovered a concept that has revolutionized our way of thinking about our compulsive overeating.

"That concept is 'abstinence.'

"Abstinence means simply three *moderate* meals a day with absolutely nothing in between. It means also no 'meals' while we're preparing a meal and no 'meals' while we're cleaning up the kitchen afterward. In other words, total abstinence from compulsive eating!

"If for medical reasons our doctor has ordered more than three meals a day, then of course we would plan accordingly and know that anything outside that plan would be breaking abstinence. Of course, black coffee, tea, water, and noncaloric beverages of any kind are the exception to between-meal nibbling.

"Just as the alcoholic must totally abstain from alcohol to remain sober, so we have found we must totally abstain from compulsive eating to maintain our own kind of sobriety. We call those who have achieved this kind of sobriety 'abstainers.'

"There are no 'musts' to any part of the OA program . . . indeed our Twelve-step program is only a suggested plan for recovery. Therefore, we aren't saying that abstinence is a 'must'. We're only passing on to you what we have learned from our own experience . . . that with 'abstinence' from compulsive eating we have at last found the true meaning of sobriety for the compulsive overeater."

In 1962 this was a brand-new idea for us. Since the word *abstain* means "to stay away from," it seemed clear that to be abstinent in OA meant to stay away from compulsive overeating. How to do this? Since we must eat, the most logical method would be to eat only at mealtimes: That meant three moderate meals a day, more if health needs required them, and absolutely nothing in between.

Unfortunately, over time abstinence took on a new meaning, a corruption of the original. Instead of implying "to stay away from," it came to suggest the eating plan itself.

"What's your abstinence?" one member would ask another. What the person really meant was, "What's your eating plan?" With this confusion, it's no wonder the word *abstinence* has come to mean different things to different people.

Will the time come when we all understand that the concept of abstinence is the same for everyone . . . to stay away from compulsive overeating? Can we recognize that it is the eating plan which may be different from one person to another, perhaps different for an individual at various times in his or her life?

In 1962 my unexpected insight was difficult to grasp, even harder to put into practice. Today it is no easier, but we *can* meet the challenge. Together we can climb those Twelve Steps to recovery, abstaining from compulsive overeating one day at a time!

The Year of Abstinence Awareness

I read in my most recent copy of *Lifeline*, OA's portable and inspirational magazine, that 2013 is "The Year of Abstinence Awareness." My personal journey of abstinence up this magnificent mountain trail began 16 years ago. The path looked steep and rocky, but the promise of a rewarding view from the summit compelled me to begin the trek. I knew I would need a buddy to encourage and guide me over the rough spots, so I asked someone to sponsor me.

> Though I love my svelte body, I love the Twelve-Step program and my personal journey of discovery even more.

She told me if I wanted to be successful, I would have to do what she did. I would need a plan of action. I was going to need weighed-and-measured food; a phone; a list of names to call each day; a log book to write about my journey; and books to read when I was weary or was in need of inspiration. To prepare me, she suggested I go to at least one meeting a week and listen to others who had trudged this road before me.

After 16 years on this amazing journey, the road is still steep with many opportunities for me to lose my footing, so I still go to one beginner meeting a week, two Big Book meetings and an OA-HOW meeting. I hear many wonderful stories and learn or relearn valuable lessons that have allowed me to give away 130 pounds (59 kg) of weight and go from a size 24 to a size 4.

But believe me, though I love my svelte body, I love the Twelve-Step program and my personal journey of discovery even more. The view as I climb is magnificent, the air is pure, and I feel connected to something greater than myself. I never want to lose the joy that abstinence allows me to experience, one day at a time.

— *West Orange, New Jersey USA*

Positive Result

OA defines abstinence as "the action of refraining from compulsive eating and compulsive food behaviors while working towards or maintaining a healthy body weight. Spiritual, emotional and physical recovery is the result of living the Overeaters Anonymous Twelve-Step program."

OA's definition of abstinence is helping me to say, "I am abstinent today. Thank you, Higher Power." I'm learning to feel comfortable with this fundamental OA statement because it recognizes abstinence as a progressive, evolving experience.

When I first came to OA more than 25 years ago, I understood abstinence to be a clean and clear-cut state: I was either abstinent or I wasn't, depending on how perfectly I followed my food plan, weighed every bite, and ate no food with white flour or sugar.

I never felt I could say, "I am abstinent" because I never achieved perfect eating. Now I know that most of the time, I am eating abstinently. Most of the time, I choose to eat in a manner that means I am maintaining a healthy weight and eating nutritious meals of sane portions. I have maintained my 40-pound (18-kg) weight loss for more than 15 years. From experience I know which are my trigger foods, so I'd better stay away from them; but if I stray, that doesn't mean I am not abstinent. Abstinence means I realize I am off-track, and I move back onto the road of recovery, moving toward or maintaining a normal weight.

I use OA's tools to help me evaluate what food my body needs and what is available. I've used the tool of writing to help me keep track of what I am eating. Talking with my sponsor about my eating patterns has been very important to my recovery. Attending meetings every week and doing service by making phone calls and talking about OA literature have helped me maintain a healthy size.

Day after day I try to partner with my Higher Power to discover where I can cut back a little more. I always want more to eat than my body needs. I am always in danger of overeating.

I like this definition of abstinence because it states a positive result we get from our OA program. We each develop our own plan of eating to get this result. I also like this definition because it reflects a new way of eating, not a short-term diet. I am abstinent when I am changing my eating habits so that my weight and size stay in a normal range.

— *Claremont, California USA*

Reaching for the Promises

Thinner is better, right? Recently I celebrated two years of abstinence, and I am maintaining a weight loss of over 100 pounds (45 kg). I thought that my considerable weight loss was an indicator that my disease was in remission. What I didn't recognize was that it had shape-shifted and was lurking in the background (sometimes even pacing in the foreground). Much of what I was calling recovery was still a manifestation of my illness. When the World Service Business Conference recently amended the abstinence definition to include compulsive eating behaviors, things came into focus for me.

My compulsive eating behaviors included the following:
- Pouring my body into the smallest-size clothing possible just for the sake of wearing that particular size regardless of whether I could breathe or sit down;
- Stepping on the scale multiple times a day, including before and after eating, before and after going to the bathroom, before and after working out—you get my drift;
- Having the perfect plan of eating (read "diet") with the perfect proportions of fat, protein, and carbs;
- Having the perfect and rigorous workout routine, adhered to religiously;
- Knowing my size in relation to yours. Was I thinner or fatter? Were you getting thinner or fatter? Did you notice I was thinner?

Was I free from the bondage of self? Heck no! Instead of feeding my face, I was feeding my ego.

So I let go of the rigid diet and punishing fitness regime. My body went up 10 pounds (5 kg), but now I'm at a weight much easier to maintain. I'm focusing on abstaining and enjoying being active. I've tossed the scale and am able to gauge how the weight is by how my clothing fits. I'm wearing a loose and comfortable size ten rather than a stiff and snug size six. I've determined that other people's weight and my own are none of my business.

Before recovery, I was reaching for the junk food. In my first year and a half of program, I was reaching for the perfect size and weight, and everyone's attention. Now I'm reaching for the promises and getting my first taste of what it means to be happy, joyous, and free.

— *Anonymous*

Quiet Reaffirmation

At first the recent change in the definition of abstinence sent a wave of worry through my brain. The old judgments surfaced: "You're not thin enough. You need to be a different size. Why don't you change your food plan?" Despite that and thanks to this program, I am no longer obese. I still hear those judgments. They try to make me forget that I enjoy physical, emotional, and spiritual recovery in this program. To combat these judgmental voices, I decided to write about "What healthy body weight means to me." The following are things I came up with:

> *To combat these judgmental voices, I decided to write about "What healthy body weight means to me."*

- wearing normal-sized clothes in small, medium, and large sizes depending on the brand (I range from sizes six to ten);
- being able to run, walk uphill, dance, exercise, jump, play sports, hike, swim, sit in a chair without worrying it will break,

and sit in an airplane seat with tray table lowered without discomfort to others or myself;
- wearing the bathing suit I bought in a "normal" store, coming out of the dressing room asking, "How do I look?" and believing the person who says, "You look great";
- having freedom from the sore knees, back, and feet that come from carrying around too much weight for my poor limbs and muscles to handle, and freedom from using a cane and walking with difficulty;
- being free of diabetes, high blood pressure, heart disease, stroke, and an increased risk of cancer because of the extra fat;
- going naked and making love without it being a gymnastic struggle in the pitch dark;
- facing sexual intimacy without feeling ashamed of my body, and trying new sexual positions with fun, laughter, and excitement;
- shopping for clothes I like, rather than clothes I think hide my fat best (which made me look huge);
- never having to go on another gosh-darned diet;
- never having to fear/hate the scale (I just weigh in at the doctor's office, and the number is about the same every time);
- loving myself and feeling my Higher Power's deep, flowing, unconditional love throughout my being;
- carrying the message of recovery through my heart, soul, mind, and body (my physical, spiritual, and emotional recovery is attractive to newcomers) and being able to say with joy, "There is a solution!" and have it sound believable.

So the next time my disease tells me I need to diet, lose weight, or be a different size, I will "quietly reaffirm" (*The Twelve Steps and Twelve Traditions of Overeaters Anonymous*, pp. 23–24) my commitment to the program principles and thank my Higher Power for my physical, emotional, and spiritual recovery saying, "Thy will, not mine, be done."

— *Anonymous*

A State of Grace

Abstinence is a state of grace by which I am balanced physically, emotionally, and spiritually. It's about food, but it's much more. It's a way of living that incorporates the principles of the Twelve Steps and gives meaning to my life. I've developed a routine that places God first in my life, and this has led to my success with abstinence. When I awake in the morning, I first say hello to my Higher Power then mentally take the first three Steps. I admit I am powerless over food and that, try as I might, I can't control my life. I remind myself that HP is restoring sanity to me. The final part of my morning ritual begins with the Third-Step Prayer from the Big Book. I conclude it by saying: "If it be Thy will, today I will follow my food plan and avoid binge foods. I will do something nice for someone today, and I will be happy. Thy will not mine be done."

This surrender to HP and my daily commitment to abstinence have added an emotional balance to my life. Without the negative feelings caused by bingeing on sugar, I am able to sail through the day on calm waters. If old feelings of irritability, discontentment, and restlessness pop up or when food thoughts surface, I repeat program phrases to myself over and over. "Easy does it." "Just for today." Usually this does the trick, but if my distraction stays with me I write about what I'm feeling. Then I share what I have written with a sponsor and follow through with any other steps that need to be taken.

Abstinence has added a spiritual dimension to my life. My mind and heart thank HP throughout the day with affirmations such as, "Thank you for the gift of abstinence."

Abstinence is a gift from my HP. To keep my abstinence alive, I have to be constantly aware of it. I have to work my program continuously. I study the Big Book and OA materials, and I live in an "attitude of gratitude" for the miracle of Overeaters Anonymous.

— *Louisiana USA*

It's Simple and It Works

My abstinence is three meals a day. I defined it that way on purpose the first day I came to OA because I didn't want abstinence to seem like a diet and because I wanted it to be something I'd stick to. In the first few weeks of abstinence I found eating just three meals a day was much more difficult than I thought it would be. I was hungry and thought about food a lot of the time. After about a month I got used to it and found that I really looked forward to those three meals, and I enjoyed not having to think about eating in between. My abstinence became, as I've heard other OA members describe it, three meals a day with *life* in between.

Now that I've had a few more months in the program, I've begun to really appreciate having a simple three-meals-a-day abstinence. My eating isn't always perfect, nor is it always guilt-free, but the fact remains that no matter what I may have eaten for my meal, the meal has an end, and I don't eat again until the next one. This represents a major change from my eating pre-OA. Then, if I'd broken a diet even a little bit, it was an excuse for binge eating. Now my imperfect three-meals-a-day abstinence means I can finish whatever it was I had for dinner and say that's all till breakfast.

I think relapsing or breaking my abstinence would be easy for me to recognize because I feel certain that if I started eating a fourth meal I would continue until I had an undeniable, full-blown binge on my hands. I acknowledge having had a "slip" if I have a bite of something and think better of it, or if I eat a larger meal than I need to and feel guilty about it.

Weight gain is another issue entirely. I take weight gain as a sign that I need to work the program more consistently. Usually when I examine what's going on within me I discover that not only have I been eating more and more of less and less healthy foods, I've also been skipping meetings and not reading, writing, or using the telephone.

All I can do in response is footwork. My bottom-line, no-frills abstinence is a major part of that footwork. It keeps me in the program and reminds me at least three times a day that I am powerless over food. Its kept me coming back one day at a time, and I'm 22 pounds (10 kg) lighter than I was when I walked in.

— Los Angeles, California USA

Freedom of Choice

Nearly nine years ago, at my first OA meeting, I was introduced to the concept of abstinence. It took the form of enthusiastic applause from members at the mention of any length of abstinence—from day one to umpteen years. At the break, some members explained to me that abstinence was refraining from eating compulsively. That didn't mean much to me, but I kept coming back because those people had something I wanted; I just wasn't sure what it was.

> *I strongly believe that if food were my sole problem, I would not be a compulsive overeater.*

During the next four months I learned many things about our common disease, not the least of which was that one symptom is perfectionism. This is one of my most devastating character defects. As a perfectionist, I set unbearably difficult standards for myself, and just as I am about to attain them, I redefine an even more difficult standard. I learned early on, and am still convinced, that the pursuit of perfection is a wasteful, stressful preoccupation. Many members offered me some valuable insight into perfectionism, and gave excellent examples of the toll it had taken in their lives and the steps they had taken to make progress in this area.

But for many OA members there was apparently one exception to the process of becoming less of a perfectionist, and that was in regard to abstinence. I continued to hear more about abstinence at every OA meeting, but it seemed not everyone defined abstinence the same way. I heard about "perfect back-to-back" abstinence. This term received the loudest and longest applause. I also heard about "gray sheet" abstinence, "sloppy" abstinence, "human" abstinence, "moderate meal" abstinence, and abstinence qualified by a host of other adjectives. In those days there often was little if any distinction between *abstinence* and *diet*. Most troubling to me was the unspoken notion that one was worthy in the eyes of OA only if one's abstinence was "perfect." I began to see people dropping out when they broke their abstinence or if they couldn't achieve the "perfect back-to-back" variety.

The longer I'm in OA the more convinced I am that there are many paths one can successfully travel to attain the spiritual awakening mentioned in the Twelfth Step. For me, this also holds true for abstinence. At the 1988 World Service Business Conference, a statement on abstinence was adopted that read, in part, "According to the dictionary, abstinence means 'to refrain from'. In Overeaters Anonymous, abstinence means to refrain from compulsive eating . . ." This was not new to me as this was the concept I'd first heard in OA. I think nearly everyone in the program agrees that to be abstinent means that you don't eat compulsively. Where there is disagreement is in the many differing views of what compulsive eating entails. I haven't seen a definition of compulsive eating, nor do I recall any attempt by OA as a whole to address this issue.

To me, compulsive eating (or overeating) is eating to feed my disease—not my body's nutritional needs. Therefore I am abstinent when I eat to feed my body and not my disease. This concept has become my ideal of abstinence. It is a goal I can never achieve perfectly, nor do I attempt to do so. I don't imagine there is a person alive who eats strictly for nourishment at all times. To be physically abstinent I only have to follow the food plan I choose for myself each day as best as I am able.

I strongly believe that if food were my sole problem, I would not be a compulsive overeater. Why I turned to food and compulsive eating—that is the basis of my disease. Bingeing, obesity, and eating in secret are but physical manifestations of my disease, which I have come to realize is emotional and spiritual.

Emotionally, I found that my reactions to my feelings—not the feelings themselves—are important components of my disease. Everyone has feelings—that's part of being human. But my reactions to my feelings were usually childish, negative, and self-destructive, and resulted in overeating. Working this program aids my emotional recovery by showing me how to deal with my feelings in a positive, adult, self-loving way. Practicing abstinence is one way to do this.

Spiritually, I believe my compulsive overeating resulted from my building barriers to keep my Higher Power out of my life. Abstinence removes these barriers and puts me in conscious contact with my Higher Power. Perfect emotional and spiritual abstinence is not attainable, just as perfect physical abstinence is not attainable.

In OA, we are free to follow any eating plan we choose: if we need a strict, weighed and measured diet, we can have it; if we need to avoid only one specific food, that's what we do; if we need to change our whole approach because of changes in our health or any other aspect of our lives, we make that change. No one in OA disputes another's individual approach to emotional recovery, and certainly there is unquestioned tolerance regarding the choice of a Higher Power. Why, then, is there often encroachment on an individual's approach to physical recovery?

A slogan I heard at my first meeting was "progress, not perfection." I see this applying to food as to every other aspect of the OA program. The more we as a Fellowship take such an approach, the more people will recover. I'm sad to say that I've known some members who gave up on OA and themselves because they couldn't live up to someone else's concept of abstinence. Our responsibility pledge says, "Always to extend the hand and heart of OA to all who share my compulsion; for this I am responsible." It doesn't say, to all who share my food plan or Higher Power or any other aspect of life. All I need to know about a person who comes to OA is that he or she is a compulsive overeater. That tells it all.

In the Big Book story entitled, "He who loses his life," the author makes the following statement about the AA philosophy: "I have seen that there is only one law, the law of love, and there are only two sins; the first is to interfere with the growth of another human being, and the second is to interfere with one's own growth." I hope and pray that OA can adopt that philosophy as its own.

— *Overland Park, Kansas USA*

Inseparable Solution

"Write an article for *Lifeline*." I kept hearing that phrase in my head. It isn't that I hadn't thought of doing it before, but every time I decided on a topic, I'd see it in the next issue of the magazine!

But there is a subject that has been on my mind lately, and I believe that we cannot say enough about it. That is, the importance of abstinence versus the importance of recovery. Can the two be separated? Can I have one without the other? I don't believe so.

> *When food was my god, my world was very limited—emotionally, physically, and spiritually.*

I hear a lot of talk about this subject in OA in my area. For example, I'd suggested that there be an abstinence requirement for speakers at one of the meetings I go to, which brought up a lot of feelings among members, including one important question: Is the time one has been in the program more important than how much abstinence one has?

I can only speak from my own experience. Please understand that I am not trying to minimize the importance of continuing to attend meetings and of working the program to the best of one's ability even if one is not presently abstaining. I attended OA meetings for ten years before I was able to abstain on a continuous basis. Had I not kept coming back, who knows where I would be today. The real question is, how much was I able to recover while I was still practicing my disease?

At the end of Step One in the AA *Twelve Steps and Twelve Traditions*, it states, "Practicing AA's remaining eleven steps means the adoption of attitudes and actions that almost no alcoholic who is still drinking can dream of taking." Is this any less true for the compulsive overeater? I don't believe so. Isn't my recovery dependent on the adoption of certain spiritual principles, and don't I need to work the Steps to accomplish that? Yes!

My first ten years in the program were a struggle, to say the least. Yes, I did make progress, but slowly. Now, after abstaining for more than twelve years, I can see the difference between that slow progress and the real progress I have made since beginning to abstain. And the changes have been dramatic.

When food was my god, my world was very limited—emotionally, physically, and spiritually. I went to work, to the market, home, and then to bed. My relationship with my two sons consisted mostly of my yelling at them. I felt so much shame and degradation because I was not able to give them the love and nurturing they needed. I did not perform very well on my job because the obsession with food was so strong. I was not capable of a healthy relationship with a man. I really just wanted someone to love me and take care of me—someone I could control. I had no relationship with God; I was not capable of that because my disease separated me from God.

All of the above was a part of my first ten years in OA. What has changed in the last dozen years, you might ask? Well, just about everything!

Today, my sons and I have a very open relationship. The transformation began when I stopped spanking them. With that, their fear of me lessened. Then I found I could talk to them in a normal tone of voice. We started to love one another. I was also helped by several kind and loving people who pointed out the error of some of my ways. Because those people told me lovingly—and because I was not eating—I came to see what they were talking about, and thus changed my actions. I stayed abstinent through many difficult years, and I am happy to say that I and my sons, who are now eighteen and twenty years old, are now on the other side.

At one time, I was unable to perform on a job because of my obsession with food. With abstinence came an opportunity for a real career. My self-esteem had been very low in that area, but with each small success, it grew. Today, I am successful in my work. The best part is that I know I am good at what I do, and that I am capable and intelligent. I look and act professionally because I am a professional.

Today, my husband and I have a relationship that I never dreamed was possible or thought I deserved. Six years ago we separated, and all my closest friends thought we were headed for the divorce court. They believed there was no way that our relationship could survive. But we worked hard to make it good, and it has paid off. I abstained through it all. What a miracle.

The biggest change of all—without which I don't believe any of the others would have been possible—is my relationship with God. I know that as long as I make food or any other person, place, or thing my god, I leave no room for a loving Higher Power in my life.

The greatest gift of my abstinence is the feeling I have knowing that my life is directed by God. It is only in retrospect that I can see how God works in my life. Whenever I have a problem or a situation that causes me discomfort, I look back over the years and remind myself that, with God in charge, everything always works out for good, even if I cannot see it at the time.

The Big Book says that we have a daily reprieve based upon the maintenance of our spiritual condition. I have experienced that reprieve because I have been rescued from a deadly disease, one that could surely kill me. I owe my life to God for providing the rescue and for continually showing me the way.

So, how important is my recovery if I am not abstaining? For me, I cannot have one without the other.

— *San Rafael, California USA*

Perplexed About Abstinence?

My first OA sponsor had me write a food history when I first came into OA. I recounted everything I could remember about my lifelong relationship to food. This included when, where, and why I ate; eating buddies; binge "sites," such as restaurants and favorite rooms in the house; trigger emotions and trigger foods.

The idea of "trigger foods" was new to me. As I thought about my life in the food, I began to see patterns. By the end of the food history, I had a list of foods that were my main choices when I wanted to binge. I used this list to identify foods from which I needed to abstain. I find that abstaining from my trigger or binge foods (as well as trigger places and situations) makes it easier to be abstinent, because I am not activating my compulsion to overeat.

My list changes over time. Some foods that I could eat early in my abstinence make me crazy now. Other foods I can eat with no problem sometimes, but get obsessive about at other times. I try to gauge whether I can handle them on a particular day. Within seconds of tasting some foods I know I will never be able to eat them sanely. They give me the crazies, taste too good, or have me obsessing about when I can have them again. When this happens, I usually pray about it, talk to my sponsor, and commit to not eating that food today. My current list of problem foods is longer and more comprehensive than it was when I first made it, but I have heard from people with long-term abstinence that "the road gets narrower."

This is not just about discipline or weight loss. It is about survival. The Big Book tells me, and I believe it with all my heart, that I have a mental obsession and a physical craving. When activated, the mental obsession and physical craving are sheer hell. For today, I will do what I must to avoid them. The temporary pleasure of eating a food that tastes good, that brings back memories of old times, or that my friends enjoy isn't worth the risk. Give me abstinence with peace of mind.

I hope this is helpful to newcomers who may find all the talk in meetings about abstinence, food plans, binge foods, flour, and sugar perplexing. Our abstinence is all the same. We don't eat compulsively, one day at a time, but our food plans differ widely. You may or may not be able to eat what I eat and stay abstinent. Writing a food history helped me identify my problem areas so I could ask for help and develop a food plan that was healthy for my body and mind. Maybe this method will work for you, too.

— *Fairfax, Virginia USA*

Say Yes to Abstinence

I've been in program three years. One day at a time, for the last three months, I've been gaining the gift of abstinence. I've lost 24 pounds (11 kg). I like to think that instead of saying no to extra food, I'm saying yes to God's gift of abstinence. What a difference that focus makes! When I serve myself healthy-sized portions of food with the nutrients my body needs, I'm feeding my body, soul, and spirit. When I eat more than my body needs, I harm myself—body, soul, and spirit.

> *I gain clarity of mind to work the Twelve Steps and get on with my life.*

This disease tells me I'm denying myself something tasty and soothing. What a *lie!* Sure it will taste good, but as soon as I stop eating, discomfort, guilt, and distance from my Higher Power follow. I will have said no to God's gift of abstinence.

So what do I gain when I say yes to abstinence? I gain clarity of mind to work the Twelve Steps and get on with my life. I can face the problems that sent me to food for comfort, and change what I can and accept the rest. I'm learning to accept that I'll often feel like I'm saying no to the "good things" others enjoy.

Feelings aren't facts, though. When I feel that way, I have tools I can pick up to work through my feelings. I can reach out to someone else; write about my feelings; tell God about my feelings; and work my recovery by choosing abstinence, one day at a time. I'd rather say yes to abstinence!

— *Savannah, Georgia USA*

CHAPTER TWO

Practical Ways to Achieve Abstinence

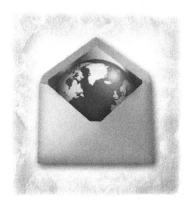

Food Corral

I am gratefully celebrating eight years of continuous abstinence. When I joined OA, I met a woman who said something astounding: she had abstained from sugar for several years. It was as if she had said she hadn't breathed for years. Sugar was my main drug to make me happy, to calm me down, to pump me up. It successfully did those things for a while. But as time went on, I needed more and more sugar to get the same effect. My life problems kept mounting, as did my fear of facing them. My life started spinning out of control.

> *How do you get and stay abstinent, especially when you want to eat compulsively more than anything?*

When I came to OA, abstinence confused me. What is it? How do you know if you are abstinent? How do you get and stay abstinent, especially when you want to eat compulsively more than anything?

Fortunately, I met a sponsor who could answer my questions. She told me to make a "food corral"—to draw a circle on a piece of paper and write inside the circle the foods and eating behaviors that caused me problems. She told me that as long as I stayed outside the corral, I was abstinent.

I made my corral and wrote inside it the foods that hurt me physically, giving me a headache or stomachache. I wrote the foods that I couldn't eat in moderation, that "owned me" after I ate just one, creating a craving for more. I also listed eating behaviors that tripped me up: overeating at buffet restaurants, grocery shopping when I was ravenous, and eating late at night.

I hated making that corral! It meant I had to get honest about foods I couldn't eat. It meant I couldn't binge anymore or convince myself it was okay. Once I put these things on paper, I knew what I needed to do and had no more excuses.

It wasn't easy. Many times I had to pick up that 2,000-pound telephone and ask for help. I knew that I would binge and have to start again if I did not reach out.

I've revised my food corral many times. I started with a small list of problem foods and kept adding to it as I got more honest. I still revise my corral. Recently, I had to change my food plan for medical reasons. I again wrote down what abstinence was for me and committed it to my sponsor.

I know that I never have to eat compulsively again as long as I work the OA program and stay away from that first compulsive bite. I have a food corral that I don't enter. Instead, I let God guide me. After eight years of abstinence, life is challenging in many ways, but it is better than I ever dreamed possible. I am grateful to my first sponsor for showing me the way and to OA for giving me the strength to live an abstinent life, one day at a time.

— *Encinitas, California USA*

Building the Foundation

I heard the words each week at the beginning of our meeting: "Abstinence is the foundation of our program." It took months for that phrase to sink into my food-fogged mind as I kept trying to find a way to work the Steps while still eating my favorite binge foods. My efforts at moderation led to a weekend-long binge that left me a physical and emotional wreck. At last a light bulb clicked on. I had to take abstinence seriously. It's not just an important part of the OA program; it's essential. Abstinence is the foundation of our program.

> *Abstinence is the foundation of our program.*

What does foundation mean? My dictionary offers several definitions, including "a basis upon which something stands or is supported" and "ground upon which something is built up." If I wanted recovery, I would have to build it on a solid foundation of abstinence. Without abstinence, my recovery would crumble (as I had already learned) or be knocked flat by any emotional storm that blew through my life.

So four months after I came to OA, I found a sponsor and committed to abstinence and a plan of eating. I did a Step-One inventory of my favorite binge foods and binge-eating situations, and I surrendered them all to God. I started planning my food each morning and emailing it to my sponsor. Those first days of abstinence were difficult, even painful. My cravings were intense. I suffered headaches during the day, and at night I dreamed about the sugary foods that had once been my constant companions. But with the support of my sponsor, I made it through those white-knuckle times and abstinence gradually became easier.

At first it was a gift I gave myself, and something I had to work at. Now, 107 days later, abstinence is a gift I receive from God. On most days it's effortless. I renew my commitment each morning in prayer: "God, please help me to be abstinent today, no matter what." Then I pray the first three Steps: "I admit I am powerless over food, that my life can become unmanageable. I have come to believe you can restore me to sanity. I now make a conscious decision to turn my life and my will over to you." I conclude with "Thank you, God, for all the blessings and miracles in my life and for all the blessings and miracles to come."

After those prayers, I open my eyes feeling clear-headed, hopeful and, best of all, sane. I've discovered abstinence makes it easier to work the Steps with honesty and to face my emotions and character defects. I'm also experiencing the benefits of physical recovery, including 27 pounds (12 kg) released, increased energy, and peaceful sleep. I still have blue days and bad moods, but I've learned to pick up the phone instead of the food. Experience has taught me I have no hope of recovering unless I'm abstinent and no hope of staying abstinent unless I'm recovering by working the Twelve Steps.

Abstinence has become the foundation of my program.

— *Eagan, Minnesota USA*

Step One Situation

Since I have been in program, I have struggled with abstinence a few times, but most days I am blessed with a solid abstinence. Most of this is because of the support of working the OA Twelve-Step program to the best of my ability. I rely on Twelve-Step literature. My literature often has kept me aware so that I don't binge.

During my sixteen years in OA, of all of the Steps I've experienced, Step One has played a huge role in maintaining my abstinence. "We admitted we were powerless over food—that our lives had become unmanageable." Writing this inspires me!

> *Step One has played a huge role in maintaining my abstinence.*

I am powerless over more than just food in my life. I am powerless over how things happen at work, over behaviors of family and friends, over how our pets act. Before I walked into these rooms, I would be unladylike with my choice of words and actions; often I would binge and overeat my many trigger foods.

Today when I find my life in a Step One situation, I find the true blessing of OA. I don't have to choose to binge, use a laxative, or compulsively overeat. I can feel what may be an unhappy part of my life and deal with it to make it better. I do this by using my Twelve-Step literature, admitting I am powerless over the situation, and taking care of myself.

How? I eat healthier food. I may go to a face-to-face or telephone meeting. Perhaps I share with my sponsor, sponsee, or an online OA loop. Until I recognize, accept, and admit that the situation is Step One and I am powerless, I cannot act. My blessing is that I no longer need to eat over it. By working Step One in many aspects of life, I keep my abstinence intact.

As far as keeping my abstinence with a support system, that would be my sponsor, sponsees, other OA members, family, and friends. My daughter, granddaughters, husband, son, music teacher, and many co-workers have often encouraged me not to give up through the years. They remind me how much I work my program when I am in a "normal" state of mind. They encourage me by letting me know that often my strength has kept them going in different situations. I am often inspired by their patience or when they hand me my Twelve-Step books, be it a *Lifeline* magazine or the Big Book.

Without Step One and the support of all these people in my life, in honesty I am not sure I would have the abstinence that has blessed me for these sixteen years in the OA program.

— Erie, Pennsylvania USA

What Is a Healthy Weight?

Having been a professional yo-yo dieter, the hardest thing has been learning and accepting the amount of food and exercise my body needs to stay around the same weight permanently.

What is a healthy weight anyway? When I was 50 pounds (23 kg) overweight, I said I was a "healthy" weight, but it was a lie. My anorexic side is never satisfied with how thin I am, so I struggle with deciding what is a healthy weight.

I have come to rely on fellow OA members and height-and-weight charts to tell me if I am healthy. I am 5 feet 4 inches (163 cm) tall and stay around 130 pounds (59 kg). At age 40, that seems to be a healthy weight for me. I still don't like it. I'd rather be 125 (57 kg) or less, but I've been there and didn't look or feel healthy.

When I weigh over 135 pounds (61 kg), I feel fat and lethargic. I weigh once a month to stay honest about my weight. When I see the weight creeping up, I know it's time to inventory my food and start cutting back a little. I do not restrict my food or take second helpings. I don't eat sweets because I'm more powerless over the craving once sweets are in my system. I eat real food—just in smaller quantities. I am able to attend picnics and eat in restaurants because I have a plan for what I'll eat, and I ask God for the strength to stick with it as imperfectly as I can. I have learned to focus on the people around me, not on how much food I can eat.

To maintain my abstinence at work, I eat my breakfast before I go, and I pack lunch and eat it (it's easy to pack lunch and then conveniently go out for lunch thinking I'll keep my packed lunch for tomorrow). Most of my co-workers know I'm an OA member, and they respect my limitations because they know I'm serious about my program. They don't push food on me. I always say, "No, thank you."

Sometimes when I start feeling sorry for myself because I won't eat something sitting around, I take one, wrap it in a paper towel, crush it and throw it away. This helps me feel like I had my share and have strangled the disease with my bare hands!

The hardest thing at work is office meetings. The company buys lunch for everyone, and everyone eats during the meeting. I could participate if the meeting time coincided with my lunch time, but it does not. My co-workers are still eating three hours after I've had lunch and three hours before it's time for my dinner. Since I eat three meals a day with nothing in between, I am unable to eat with them because it is not time to eat.

If the smell of food gets too overwhelming, I pop a sugar-free mint in my mouth, and I always have my water. If the eating meeting disturbs me too much, I call an OA member or go to a meeting after work to help me cope.

— *Woodsboro, Maryland USA*

In the Field

As an anorexic compulsive eater, I follow a rigid food plan in quantity and eating times. This often works well to remove the cause of my obsession, if I've eaten the right amount. I define abstinence as "doing what's best for me." This sometimes conflicts with my food plan.

My job as a lecturer is sedentary, but about three times a year I take students out for a fieldwork day. This involves carrying heavy equipment over rough ground, running along the survey line to instruct students or to drive away inquisitive animals, and hammering the ground with a sledgehammer to create seismic vibrations. I may also drive for the first time in months (I don't own a car).

Before OA I was on a field trip sitting on a quarry rock in tears; I had run out of energy. I had brought even less food than I would eat on a non-fieldwork day! On later field trips, I brought a candy bar, but it filled my head before my stomach. I took extra lunch food, then almost fell asleep while driving a minibus full of students. It has taken me 10 years in OA to realize the hard part of fieldwork is the early part: loading equipment, surveying the site, and setting out instruments. So a larger breakfast and a mid-morning snack are the keys to an abstinent day.

Flexibility about when to eat and assertiveness in saying I will eat *now* are essential. When my food's wrong, I get tired, dictatorial, and careless; the many little problems of fieldwork frustrate me. Having eaten appropriately, I give myself the chance to be patient, strong, encouraging, and even scientifically inspired—in short, to do my job properly. It is good for me to write this for people who understand just what a miracle this recovery is.

— *Birmingham, United Kingdom*

Relapse Prevention

I've been abstaining in OA for over eleven years, maintaining a 110-pound (50-kg) weight loss for ten of them. Although none of us is cured and there's always the threat of relapse, the miracle of OA is that relapse is not inevitable. OA has given me and countless others a way of life that works.

When I first got abstinent, I was scared of relapse. My life before OA had been one of constant "relapse" with a few transitory stretches of almost successful dieting. At last I'd found something that seemed to work, and I was scared of people in relapse, afraid that

> *One of the most common precursors to relapse is insufficient attendance at OA meetings.*

their troubles with food might be contagious and lead me back to destructive eating.

As my sponsor wisely pointed out, however, I didn't have to worry about catching the disease of compulsive overeating—I already had it.

My sponsor pointed out that in OA we recover by working with other compulsive overeaters, and that includes those in relapse. He suggested that working closely with these people would help me learn from their mistakes without having to repeat them myself.

What are some of those mistakes? One of the most common precursors to relapse is insufficient attendance at OA meetings. It's been my observation that those who attend frequently and do service seem to relapse less than those who attend infrequently. Sometimes we've come so far that we think we're cured and no longer need OA meetings.

Other common mistakes involve not using one or more of the tools, or not working all of the Steps. A person might try to get by without a commitment to a service position or without writing a Fourth-Step inventory. Working all the Steps and using all the tools doesn't mean a life without food problems, but not working the program will guarantee them.

To watch a close OA friend go through this painful experience is distressing. A relapse takes on a life of its own, with temporary moments of hope followed by painful demoralization. Sometimes it seems as if nothing will end it. But relapses burn themselves out sooner or later. They may end faster for those who attend lots of OA meetings, but they never end quickly enough.

I admit that I'm powerless over food—and that includes other people's food as well. There's nothing I can do to guarantee that others will stay abstinent, but I can pray for them, talk to them, and offer rides to meetings. I try not to offer advice unless asked, since I know how I hate it when others give it to me.

Here's what I do to stay abstinent: Every morning, I ask God for help, and then take a few moments of quiet time and meditate. I call my sponsor almost every day, and I sponsor several people.

I attend about five OA meetings a week. It's easy for me to eat properly when I get to a lot of meetings and harder when I don't. I have a service position at a meeting, which makes it more likely that I'll show up. My phone calling, reading, and writing are more sporadic, but over the course of a month I'll use all the tools.

I eat the same number of meals a day, and I pay close attention to portion size. I don't eat foods that cause problems for me, including some that others in program are able to handle.

At night I do a mental Tenth-Step inventory and remind myself that my disease is threefold: physical, emotional, and spiritual. I then ask myself where I am physically, emotionally, and spiritually to identify what areas in my life need attention.

I keep a big margin of safety in my program. I don't ever want to return to the living hell of compulsive overeating and morbid obesity.

— *Arlington, Virginia USA*

Condition Check

I've heard people speak about sloppy abstinence ever since I've been in the OA program. I never cared much for that term. I felt that if one set down a plan of abstinence, one either stuck to it or one didn't. Certainly that was the case for me.

Now my abstinence has gotten sloppy. I haven't relapsed, but there's a real risk of my doing just that. Suddenly I realize that I have to eat some of my own words—and they're not on my food plan!

I've come face-to-face with my powerlessness. I don't want to admit to myself that I'm still powerless. I've been in program for several years now, and I should be getting it right. I haven't been doing the things I said I wouldn't do with my eating, and thus haven't specifically broken my abstinence. Still the obsession with food has been sneaking back in.

I always expected that relapse, if it came, would come with a crash—but instead it appears to be creeping in, little by little. In a way, that's good—with God's help, I can stop it before it gets out of hand, but a "creeping" relapse may be more difficult to recognize.

After the discussion of Step Ten in the Big Book (page 84), it says, "by this time sanity will have returned . . . If tempted, we recoil . . . as from a hot flame. We react sanely and normally, and we will find that this has happened automatically." This promise was granted to me for a long time, but lately I've found that more often than not it hasn't been the case.

Why was this promise fulfilled in my life and then, to a degree at least, taken from me? I find the answer in the next paragraph. "We are not cured . . . What we really have is a daily reprieve contingent on the maintenance of our spiritual condition." Clearly my spiritual condition must be lacking.

I've looked at the things I did when I first came into the program and what I'm doing now, and I notice that I've selectively stopped doing some of those things. For instance, I used to pray regularly; I now pray intermittently. I learned to meditate and now rarely do. I was strict with my food plan and my abstinence; I'm now much looser. I exercised regularly; I don't any longer. I wrote daily; lately, it's several times a month. I used to read program literature every day; now I do it when I get the time, maybe once every week or two. I suppose what I'm realizing is that these efforts aren't sufficient for me to remain in fit spiritual condition.

I tend to see things in black-and-white terms: I'm either abstinent or I'm not; I'm either working my program or I'm not. This is false. I'm still abstinent by my own definition, even though my abstinence hasn't been as clean as I'd like. I've been working my program, but not to the degree that I need to.

I'm still sponsoring and doing lots of service, and I'm of some help to those who still suffer. I'm still reading literature, making phone calls, writing, and getting to a good many meetings. So where do I go from here?

I met with my sponsor and wrote out a plan of action that I felt would help me. It set reasonable goals for me to work toward, specifically in the areas of food plans, writing, reading, meditation, and exercise. My sponsor also suggested a couple of other areas to work on that I hadn't thought of. He emphasized to me that whatever happens now, and whether or not I accomplish it, is totally up to God.

First, I must surrender completely to God. Then I need to do what I can to regain my fit spiritual condition.

I look forward to getting back into that place where I can feel good about myself and get back to losing weight. When and if I do, the credit will go to God, my Higher Power.

— *San Antonio, Texas USA*

Plugging the Dam

Three weeks ago I found myself in relapse again. My eating was out of control and I felt as if I were drowning in food. The scariest part was that I had no idea when or why it started. I didn't make a conscious decision to start using the food again; it just happened. But I'd stopped doing my footwork and I hadn't been to an OA meeting in a month due to a vacation—and cockiness. My abstinence had been going so well—what did I need a meeting for?

> *Now I know that the "controlled eating" of "just one" leads to the uncontrolled eating of many more.*

What I did was like taking my finger out of a hole in a dam. The hole got bigger and bigger as I decided it was okay to eat certain foods that weren't a part of my abstinence; in other words, my binge foods. Eventually the dam burst, and I was awash in food.

The sick part of my brain took over. I had trouble remembering that I had a disease. If I could eat "just one" of a certain binge food, my thinking went, then surely I was a normal eater. Now I know that the "controlled eating" of "just one" leads to the uncontrolled eating of many more. Eventually my abstinence is gone and I'm back into my illness.

This relapse scared me enough to examine why I couldn't or wouldn't turn my abstinence and program over to my Higher Power.

I asked myself: "What have I got to lose by believing that a power greater than myself can take my food addiction and restore me to sanity?" My answer: I'd lose the food, how I wanted to eat it, and when.

I realized then just how strong my illness is. I wasn't willing to give up the food and had decided that I wouldn't like the new life my HP would make for me. I understood how sick it was to decide I didn't want to be restored to sanity and abstinence because I thought I knew what the outcome would be. In reality I have no idea what recovery will be like. I know it can't be worse than the pain and insanity of this last relapse.

I prayed for willingness and decided I had nothing to lose—except excess food—by believing my HP could and would restore me to sanity. I became willing to make daily food plans and call them in to my food sponsor.

At this point I'd been in OA a year and had never been willing to call in my food before. I enjoyed deciding what I wanted to eat right before my meals. I realized that I'd gotten a lot of excitement from eating what I wanted right at the moment, but the willingness to call in my food came from my HP.

This has been a hard year. After my first seven days of abstinence I remembered that I'd been an incest victim as a child. For a long time I used my pain as an excuse to overeat, with the rationale that I had to use anything I could to get through these painful, fearful days.

Reading "Journey Through Deception" in the Brown Book helped me more than I can say. It taught me that, if I want to get well, I can't use the pain of my childhood as an excuse to overeat. Food doesn't help the pain—it buries it. To recover, I must feel all of my feelings; to do that, I must be abstinent.

I'm willing to go to any length to remain abstinent. I'm going to OA meetings, reading OA literature every day, and talking with my food sponsor every night. I'm still scared of relapse, so I'm praying to my HP and continuing to turn my will and my life over every day.

— *Athens, Georgia USA*

Travel Insurance

I love to travel and am blessed to have the opportunity to take many trips each year. Because I am a compulsive overeater, however, traveling offers me extra challenges on the road to recovery. In the past, a trip had been an excuse to overeat, and I often gained large amounts of weight while away from home. But since working the OA program of recovery, I can travel and maintain my abstinence and weight. I would like to share some of the methods that have worked for me.

- Get meeting lists and contact members. Long before I leave home, I write to the World Service Office to obtain a list of meetings and contacts for the area I'm visiting. It's always gratifying to see the program in action in other places and to feel the familiar OA warmth in an unfamiliar area.
- Find out what the "food scene" will be like ahead of time. If it's a business meeting I'm going to, I call to ask whether preset breakfasts or lunches will be included, and, if so, what foods will be served. If I'm visiting a friend, I politely but honestly make my food needs known before I arrive. After getting as much information as I can, I make up a food plan with my sponsor. Sometimes this plan includes a commitment to eat a little differently than I would at home.
- Plan ahead for airline travel. Before I fly, I carefully think through my meals. I almost always bring my own lunch, and sometimes my own supper. That way I'm assured I'll eat foods that are healthy for me. If there are delays, I can still eat my meals at regular times.
- If possible, prepare your own meals. On vacations, my husband and I try to stay at places that have kitchens. That way, we can have breakfast "at home" and take a picnic lunch with us. Besides helping me stay abstinent and avoid so many restaurant meals, it's fun!
- Take program literature along. I take a supply of OA literature with me, especially *Lifeline*, because it's small and easy to pack.

- Keep in touch with your sponsor. My sponsor has received calls from many faraway places! Sometimes we set a telephone date so I can be sure to reach her.
- Keep a food journal. While traveling, I write down what I eat and any feelings I may be having about my food. When I get home, I give this journal to my sponsor to read. I like knowing that someone will know how I ate—both on the days that I felt good about my food and on the days I felt shaky.
- Be flexible. And that brings me to the last but possibly most important aspect of traveling abstinently: remember to be flexible—accept food situations that are beyond one's control. I need to be extra kind and, above all, forgiving of myself if I eat differently than I'd eat at home.

OA teaches me to live in the world. Although I can never forget that I have the disease of compulsive overeating, I've found that I can experience the joys of traveling as I continue to recover.

— *Chapel Hill, North Carolina USA*

Crystal Clear

Last year we had a family get-together in Sacramento and went to the zoo and the museum. We had a picnic lunch in the park and my mother-in-law brought some cupcakes. I didn't have one, but after everyone else ate all they wanted, there were several left over. She gave them to me, and I quickly bundled them into the car.

The next day during the trip home, I noticed them and offered them to the kids to finish off. I wanted one (or ten) quite a bit, so I was relieved to see them all eaten up—or so I thought.

My youngest ate about half of his, including the icing, then gripping it in his hand for a while, he fell asleep in his car seat. The cupcake fell on the floor of the car. When we stopped to stretch a couple of hours later, I helped him out of his car seat and picked up the half-eaten, dirty, stale cupcake. Instead of throwing it away as I had meant to, I stuffed it into my mouth.

When I told an OA friend this story to illustrate how sick I continue to be, she told me about a very expensive and beautiful crystal bowl she and her husband were given for a wedding present. It was too valuable to be used every day, so it was put away for special occasions.

One day, when she was dusting, she carelessly dropped a cheap ceramic bowl on it and helplessly watched her priceless crystal shatter into a thousand pieces.

She tied the two stories together—my abstinence was the precious crystal and the dirty cupcake was the ceramic bowl. Did I want to break my priceless abstinence for a piece of trash? This symbolic mental image has stuck with me and helped me through quite a few rough spots. As much as I may want to eat a particular something, it isn't worth it; my abstinence is much too valuable to me to break so carelessly.

— *Susanville, California USA*

Time-Tested Recovery

At three o'clock in the morning on the Saturday after Thanksgiving I could not get to sleep. I felt horrible because of the bingeing I had done for the previous two days, and I was scared. For some time I have been struggling emotionally with a special relationship in my life that is not going the way I had hoped. This relationship has been on my mind constantly, and I've been afraid of what the outcome will be. Feeling very powerless and frustrated, I used the holiday as an excuse to overeat.

> *When I was growing up I remember turning to food for comfort whenever I was afraid.*

I've been in the program a little over six years and am maintaining a 341-pound (155-kg) weight loss. My program is strong, but for those few days I didn't work it, nor did I trust my Higher Power. What I experienced was a major slip for me, and it brought back a flood of bad memories.

When I was growing up I remember turning to food for comfort whenever I was afraid. Since I felt inadequate, the fear of failure was ever present. I came into OA weighing 521 pounds (236 kgs); I was unemployed, divorced, and very desperate. I felt I had failed at everything in life, especially as a son, husband, and father. I did not want to live anymore but was too scared to do anything about it. It didn't take me long to realize that this program was exactly what I needed, so I surrendered myself to it.

My Higher Power and the loving, caring people in this program helped me to start facing the mountain of fear I had built up inside me without having to turn to food for sustenance. With every meeting I went to, every tool I used, every Step I worked, and every prayer I prayed, I was gaining strength and courage. The miracle of my recovery was beginning.

Food is cunning, baffling, and powerful. I turned to it over this past Thanksgiving holiday in order to cope with the fear I was feeling. It didn't help, of course, it never does—it just made a bad situation worse.

I have finally managed to turn that special relationship over to my Higher Power and will accept the outcome, whatever it is. I feel a great deal of relief and my abstinence has returned. Writing this article has helped too.

One thing that keeps getting stronger as my recovery progresses is the knowledge that no matter how much I may be hurting or how bad things may seem at times, as long as I maintain contact with my Higher Power and this beautiful program, I will be okay no matter what comes along. This has been proven to me time and time again throughout my recovery.

— *Racine, Wisconsin USA*

It's All in the Steps

I learned the importance of working the Twelve Steps of recovery—the hard way. When my first sponsor in Alcoholics Anonymous proposed that I use the Fourth and Fifth Steps to "clean house," I refused.

"I'm a Jesuit priest," I told him. "All I have ever done since I began studying for the priesthood is go to confession."

How wrong I was. I did not want to admit that my physical addiction was only a symptom of an underlying mental and spiritual illness. For five years I was a "dry drunk" with a two-step program: (1) I stopped drinking; and (2) I bragged about it. Failure to confront the exact nature of my wrongs kept me trapped in my character defects, and I simply switched from active alcoholism to compulsive overeating.

I reached the point of wanting to die. Suicide was not an option because I didn't think it would look good on my resume. Another Jesuit, a recovering alcoholic, finally sold me on the Fourth and Fifth Steps as the key to acquiring the restoration to sanity that the Second Step promises. I worked those two Steps with him and was granted a marvelous sense of belonging to the Fellowship of those who are in recovery.

Working the Fourth and Fifth Steps helped me to recognize that I was an egomaniac with an inferiority complex. In other Twelve-Step programs, I dealt with the origins of my depression and low self-esteem by sharing experience, strength, and hope with other adult children of alcoholics. On my first program anniversary, I told a friend how grateful I was that my feelings of uselessness and self-pity were beginning to disappear, even though I was still carrying around the extra 44 pounds (20 kg) I had gained while I was depressed.

I think I expected my friend to pat me on the back, tell me I didn't look so bad, and give me the latest and greatest diet she had found. Instead she said, "Go to Overeaters Anonymous. They know about compulsive overeating."

I resisted for a few weeks, but a Labor Day binge proved to me once again that it was insane for me to think that I could cure myself. Two days later I went to my first OA meeting and began working the Steps all over again with a new group of fellow sufferers. After two years I have shared a Fifth Step twice and am planning to do so again. I have lost 42 pounds (19 kg) and have taken eight inches off my waist. More importantly, I have gained some wisdom and serenity that help me to "live life on life's terms."

One of my chief convictions about the Steps is that there are many different ways to work them. After all, if we can each have a God according to our own understanding, may we not also work the Steps accordingly?

Some people like to view the Steps on a medical model: the first three are "intensive care," Steps Four to Nine are "inpatient treatment," and then we are healthy enough to work the last three Steps on our own. Others emphasize working the Steps in order. I once heard someone say that working the First Step is being in first grade, which would make those working the Twelfth Step seniors in the "school of recovery." To this way of thinking, the First Step is something that we get farther and farther away from the more we journey in recovery.

My own imperfect experience in recovery suggests that it is best for me to see how all Twelve Steps continue to work together to keep me on the path toward health and happiness. In the other models, going back to the First Step might feel like failure. We are liable to feel that we have "flunked out" of the higher grades and have been sent back to learn a lesson that we should not have forgotten, or that we are going backwards to square one, losing all the forward progress we thought we had made.

For me, it works best to think of each Step as support for all the others so that I am not ashamed or dismayed when I find that I need more of the wisdom available in the First Step in order to carry on with the ninth.

The First Step serves me as gasoline does an automobile: I draw regularly on the reservoir of acceptance of my powerlessness, but have to stop from time to time to fill up again on the insight that I will never save myself from the "bondage of self." The First Step is the foundation of all the other Steps, even when I am not conscious of the support it offers me.

Steps Two to Nine seem to me to work in pairs. For example, belief in a benevolent Higher Power (Step Two) enables me to turn myself over to the care of that Power (Step Three). A moral inventory (Step Four) enables me to admit the nature of my wrongs (Step Five). Readiness to change (Step Six) makes it possible for me to let go of my shortcomings (Step Seven). The list of those I have harmed (Step Eight) guides me in deciding how to make amends (Step Nine). As I work the initial Step in each of these pairs, I do so knowing there is a follow-through in the next Step.

The last three Steps are very special to me. Although I believe that it's best to work all the Steps in order, I do not see how I could have postponed working these last three Steps until I had finished making amends.

The Tenth Step is something I did daily from day one. It encouraged me to keep my current affairs clean while I labored to "clear away the wreckage" of my past. Similarly, I couldn't work any of the Steps in a healthy fashion without conscious contact with my Higher Power. I use each of the Steps as a topic for prayer and meditation. I know that this is a spiritual program, and every Step is spiritual if I allow the light of the Eleventh Step to fill all the rest.

The first part of the Twelfth Step seems to confirm this view for me: each Step contributes to my spiritual awakening. I didn't wait until I had finished working all the Steps before sharing my joy of recovery with others, nor do I want others to wait. As Bill W. discovered by helping Dr. Bob, carrying the message is essential to recovery. To me, everyone who shares at a meeting is working the second part of the Twelfth Step, even if all one can say is, "I need help" or "Food has me beaten again."

Understanding how the Steps work together in my recovery doesn't mean I pick and choose among them, substituting one I like for another that I don't like. Recognizing how they all work together helps me do what I need most for my recovery.

— *Syracuse, New York USA*

Formula for Living

With God's grace, I've had five and one-half years of clear and clean abstinence. For a person who couldn't go one day without bingeing for up to three hours, this is nothing less than a miracle!

Coming into the program, I accepted the First Step in its entirety. I still do. I know with all my heart that I am powerless over food, and that taking the first compulsive bite will return me to a life marked by despair, low self-esteem, poor health, and a fat body.

Even more impressive than the gift of abstinence is the fact that I now live comfortably without excess food. All the credit for that goes to the remaining eleven Steps of the Overeaters Anonymous Twelve-Step program.

For years it seemed as if I couldn't get full no matter how much I ate. I've come to see that food could never fill the void I had; it was a spiritual sustenance that I needed. By working the Steps, I've tapped into a Power that rests quietly within. Truly, it is a gift of the Twelve Steps.

Besides the Twelve Steps, another guide I live by is a little formula my sponsor taught me: $E + R = O$. The event plus my response equals the outcome.

Before my recovery began, I responded to most events by overeating. Relationships, jobs, vacations, health problems—all were dealt with by compulsive eating. And the outcome was always the same—remorse, fear, and pain.

The $E + R = O$ formula showed me that I needed to learn healthier responses to life and its events. Today, prayer is my first response to any uncertain situation in my life. That is followed by action, which may be to call a sponsor, go to a meeting, write, wait, or talk to the people involved.

When I follow the formula, I feel positive about the outcome.

Now, I resolve my problems by practicing the principles of the program and by utilizing my sponsor's formula. That isn't to say I don't have difficult times, but I do always have tools to deal with whatever life presents.

Being abstinent, thin, healthy, and full of life is a direct result of the Overeaters Anonymous program. It is teaching me to stand in the light, where the nourishment I need is always available.

— *Corona del Mar, California USA*

Aussie "How-To"

My name is K. and I'm a compulsive overeater. Although I am Australian, I attended my first OA meeting in Chicago in 1981. I had been en route to California after a stop in Europe to hook up with my sister.

Unfortunately for her (she is not a compulsive overeater), she ended up traveling with me through the last four horrific months of my compulsive overeating.

I thought of nothing but food. I was bad tempered, bossy, rude, selfish, and domineering. I was the older sister so I got away with it. On the last stage of our journey back across the United States, I put "us" on a diet. We were allowed to eat only crackers, cheese, and apples. Since I was driving the car, my sister had no choice; I simply would not stop to allow her out of the car to eat.

Years later she told me how she'd snuck into shops when we stopped for gas and would have a snack to keep from being hungry all the time.

When we reached California I started going to OA meetings again. Thank God, I got abstinent from the beginning. After eighteen continuous days of abstinence, I felt great. I was so proud of myself that the good feeling didn't leave me for months. I don't mean that it wasn't hard work or that it didn't require enormous effort and discipline on my part, but I felt good.

Initially, I used all sorts of tricks to avoid overeating. I established a strict timetable for my meals. Breakfast was at 7:00 a.m. I couldn't get up until then because I had to eat as soon as I got out of bed (most of the time I still do). Lunch was at noon. I'd start watching the clock at about 11:00 a.m., convinced I was starving, all the while praying for help. Dinner was at 5:00 p.m.—sometimes slightly later if I could force myself to cook slowly. By 8:30 p.m., I'd have to go to bed, because if I got hungry again, I didn't know if I could trust myself not to have that first compulsive bite.

Later on, when the obsession with mealtimes had passed and I would find myself thinking "food" at an inappropriate time, I'd use little tricks to postpone the act of compulsive overeating. I'd say to myself, "Well, first I'll have a cup of coffee. If I'm still hungry after that, then I can have something." Generally, by the time I made the coffee and drank it, the compulsion to eat would have passed and I'd be OK. I had a whole store of those phrases that started with the word *just.* For example: "just water the plants, take a bath, ring a friend, wash the dishes, hang out the wash." These phrases really helped me to learn self-discipline.

Another great help to me was identifying the emotions and situations which triggered my compulsion. I divided a sheet of paper into three columns, listing (1) when I felt like eating, (2) what my feelings were at the time, and (3) what kind of character defects I felt provoked the situation. For example, when I had visitors or when I attended social gatherings, I usually felt ill at ease, and I saw my character defect as self-centeredness. My list went on and on.

After I examined the list, I saw that "felt uneasy" came up in nearly every situation. From then on, whenever I thought I was hungry in a situation which made me feel uncomfortable, I would tell myself that it was not hunger I was feeling, but uneasiness. And I knew food would not cure that. Then I made a choice—either I could avoid such situations, or gradually, through working the Steps, I could improve my self-esteem and learn to handle them.

And guess what—I have been abstinent now for four continuous years. The obsession with food is gone, the compulsions are few and far between, and thanks to the OA program and OA friends, I have the tools to handle problems when they do arise. My experience has taught me never to underestimate my need for OA meetings and for contact with other members.

Best of all, when I am abstinent, I know I am much closer to God.

— *Tweed Heads South, Australia*

Finally, Abstinence

During the last nine months, I have finally reached a stable abstinence after struggling in OA recovery for more than nine years. A big part of that abstinence consists of my process of surrender, which means I plan my food for the day, write it down and read it to my sponsor. I go to any lengths to keep this commitment daily. OA members sometimes say that my abstinence and my program of recovery sound like dieting, but my plan of eating is unlike anything I experienced in my dieting days.

When I was dieting, my daily obsession was how to put the fewest possible calories into my body and rid myself of the rest through exercise. Of course, this behavior put my body into starvation mode and kept me constantly craving food, which led to bingeing. The bingeing caused feelings of profound remorse, and I restricted my diet even more. Eventually, I resorted to more severe choices to help me restrict my caloric intake, including over-the-counter and street drugs, diuretics, laxatives, cigarettes, and caffeine. My disease took me down a painful spiral of futility, helplessness, hopelessness, despair, and anguish.

Today, thanks to the OA program and my Higher Power, I don't live that way. I follow a plan of eating prescribed to me by a professional. I have tried to follow a plan of eating I devised myself, but I learned slowly and painfully that my disease ruled my attempts to dictate what I needed to be eating. Other food plans have caused me problems because they allowed "free foods" (which triggered my addiction to volume) or they allowed me my binge foods (which kept me in the phenomenon of craving).

Because volume is a problem for me (meaning I can binge on anything, including raw vegetables), an important part of my plan of eating is weighing and measuring portions. By weighing and measuring, I surrender the amount I'm eating. Likewise, my plan of eating has removed my binge foods, which allows me the miracle of a craving-free life.

I've had to let go of some former behaviors to follow this plan of eating. I can no longer eat spontaneously. It is more trouble and feels much more slippery to me to try to eat out than it is to prepare meals myself. Parties and dinners, while possible, are somewhat stressful and usually involve embarrassing questions that I can never seem to answer adequately. Also, I plan and pack my meals each day, which takes time and effort. However, when I plan my food, commit it and live my day without thinking about it, it is almost as if the food takes care of itself.

To stay sane and spiritually connected, I must work a rigorously honest program of recovery. Meetings, daily contact, prayer, meditation and Step work are essential for maintaining my abstinence. I always remember that my food plan would be just another diet and I'd be unable to maintain it without working my OA program. In this way, God and the OA program have restored me to sanity.

Today, working my program feels easy, and I'm grateful for the ease and comfort from which my abstinence springs. God willing, I need not diet ever again, one day at a time.

— *Anonymous*

Abstinent in Pastry Hell

A perk of my new job is that my company sent me to Paris for training. My well-meaning relatives and friends showered me with advice about how to control my eating while still sampling the local delicacies (most of which I don't eat on my current abstinence). I panicked about maintaining my abstinence in the midst of "pastry hell." Luckily, my time in program and discussions with my sponsor helped me develop a plan for staying abstinent. I left home with abstinent foods in my suitcase and a meeting list.

> OA and the Twelve Steps are a universal language.

The first thing I did was to find an English-speaking OA meeting. When I walked into that first meeting, the feeling that I was home washed over me. I felt instant fellowship. My new friends talked of recovery, abstinence, the Twelve Steps, living one day at a time, God, the lack of newcomers, relationships—all the things we discuss in my home groups. They welcomed me with open arms and shared their programs, homes, and food. The best meal I had was the abstinent meal I shared with another OA member at his home. I called these people when I needed support, and they said the same things my friends at home would have said.

Because of this Fellowship and the kindness of the people I met, I returned to the US with excess weight only in my luggage. OA and the Twelve Steps are a universal language.

— *Los Angeles, California USA*

Gift of Abstinence

The last holiday season was my first abstinent one. It was also the most enjoyable, largely because of the recovery rules I instituted to protect my abstinence. Here are my rules.

- I have $xxx to spend on the holidays. This includes gifts, cards, holiday food, wrapping, everything. I will not spend money I don't have for gifts people don't want. I will give tokens of my love and lots of cards. Overspending is stress, and stress leads to overeating. I will tell everyone that I'm not buying gifts this year. I am giving them and myself the freedom of not going into debt.
- If someone buys me a gift, I will say "thank you" without apologizing for not having one for him or her. Instead, I will give that person the gift of seeing how much I appreciate his or her thoughtfulness.
- I will not allow nonabstinent food in my living area. I will ask my family members to keep such food in the nonabstinent closet, the lower refrigerator shelves or their own rooms. My home is my refuge, and I don't need to be exposed to food pornography.
- I will not force myself to be in the presence of food that makes

me uncomfortable. If I feel fine while others indulge in holiday treats, that's wonderful. But if I feel "iffy," I will leave for a while. I won't make a fuss; I just need "fresh air."
- I will arrive late to parties and leave early. I will not overextend myself.
- I will say no to a party or gathering when I don't feel strong in my program.
- I will bring abstinent food to every holiday gathering with plenty to share.
- If someone offers me nonabstinent food, I will not go into lengthy explanations. I will just say, "No thank you; I'm not hungry right now."
- I will not drink alcohol because it lowers my defenses against food. I will be the designated driver for those I love.
- I will keep my exercise routine during the holidays—a living amends I make to myself.
- I will keep healthy and abstinent snacks stocked in my fridge and pantry at all times.
- I will enjoy my friends and family this holiday season. Holidays are not to celebrate food; food is used to celebrate the holidays. I give myself the gift of freedom from eating unhealthy food.

— *Anonymous*

You Can Too

When I first came to OA, abstinence eluded me. I didn't know it had to do with what I was not doing. I was not willing to go to any lengths to put down the food.

I came back to the food, saw misery, and it conquered me. I reached another rock bottom and this time received the gift of desperation. I knew I could not continue this way; I was willing to do whatever it took to get abstinent.

The Big Book says, "Half measures availed us nothing" (*Alcoholics*

Anonymous, 4th ed., p. 59). How true this turned out to be. What did I do to get abstinent after one and a half years in OA? I went to ninety meetings in ninety days. I got a sponsor and started working the Steps. I admitted I was a compulsive overeater and food addict. I followed my food plan and stayed away from the first compulsive bite. I handed my food over to my sponsor each day. I did service by calling newcomers and OA members and by helping out at meetings. I read OA literature and the Big Book. Each day I prayed to God for the gift of abstinence. I put my abstinence first, as the most important thing in my life without exception. I weighed and measured my food. I listened to others who had strong recovery. When the compulsion to eat came up, I took action. I said the Serenity Prayer, made a phone call, attended a meeting, or undertook a distracting activity. I got through the early days of abstinence by focusing on not picking up just for today and by using the slogans "This too shall pass" and "One day at a time." When I became willing to take these actions, I surrendered the food to God and took Step Three. God gave me the gift of abstinence. It gets much easier the longer I'm abstinent.

When I put my head on the pillow at night, as long as I've had an abstinent day, I've had a good day. Also, since I've been abstaining from sugar and simple carbohydrates, my cravings have disappeared. By the grace of God, OA and actions taken, I have been abstinent since November 29, 2006. I am now at a healthy weight. I was a food addict who could not stop bingeing, purging, or self-harming. I never thought I'd get abstinent. I thought I was finished. I will always be a food addict, and I need to work a strong program one day at a time.

I need God and you, the Fellowship of OA, because I cannot do it alone. If I could get abstinent when I was suicidal, hopeless, and desperate, then you can too.

— *Sydney, Australia*

CHAPTER THREE

The Search for Abstinence

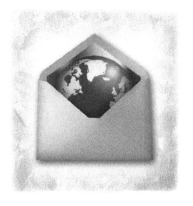

Perfect Shift

On Christmas Day 2001, I celebrated one year of abstinence. My group had supported my upcoming medallion, and urged me to celebrate my abstinence milestone at a meeting. The idea troubled me because I was terrified I would lose my abstinence over it. I had never been able to give up any of my trigger foods in the past, and here I was a year without them. Was it too good to be true? Would sharing it with the group somehow sabotage me? I had spoken with other members who understood where I was coming from. My sponsor felt I had recovery to share and urged me to accept my medallion with the group. I was confused.

I had another issue in sharing with the group. Even though I was celebrating a sustained 25-pound (11-kg) weight loss, I still felt I had not achieved true abstinence. Did I deserve to say I had been abstinent for a year when I still felt physical recovery was not mine? Because my physical recovery wasn't perfect, I didn't want to give newcomers and other members the wrong impression of recovery. With all these emotions and thoughts spinning around inside me, I had a lot of writing and praying to do too.

Over the Christmas holiday, I experienced what I like to call a shift. I've had them before, and it is how God takes me to the next level in my program. Shifts are exciting; I never know when they will come. This shift gave me the gift of consciousness in my eating. OA had given me the gift of consciousness in so many areas of my life, but I had never let it carry over into my evening mealtime. All of a sudden, I realized I had not allowed my eating to take place in a caring manner. I was not letting God guide my mood, food, or body. I began to realize I needed to slow everything down, from coming home in a starving frenzy to make food decisions, determining amounts, and actually eating.

It has been less than a week since this shift has come about, but I am amazed how I am listening to God at mealtime. One day at a time, if I continue to listen and do the footwork, I know that God will do what is best for me. He also thinks it is time for me to share my recovery.

— *Anonymous*

A Misguided Goal

Abstinence was my number one goal the first two and a half years in program. I listened to members speak glowingly about staying abstinent and about what it had done for them. I wanted that! Unfortunately, my abstinence was elusive and fleeting. I would have it for several days, only to watch my abstinence dissipate. Was I doing something wrong?

Food addiction was a difficult concept. I could not completely give up food, so it was difficult to find and keep abstinence. If only I could come to OA, stop eating and then begin to work program, as they do in AA. However, that does not happen. I felt if I was not abstinent, then I must not be working program. Such a vicious cycle!

It's too bad we can't bottle hindsight and sell it to newcomers who walk through the door. Hmm, we don't need to bottle it because I can share with you what I've learned. What did I learn through my trials and tribulations of working a Twelve-Step program for over two years before finding good recovery?

In my heart, I know my goal of abstinence was one of self-will. I wanted it, felt I should have it and felt others expected it of me. But it was not in my power because I was relying solely on my willpower. I still wanted to call the shots and control everything. I wanted program *my* way.

Fortunately, the program of Overeaters Anonymous is much better than my program. I used the tools and answered the questions from the OA workbook, but I did not implement the Steps in my life; I just gave lip service to them. Only when I shifted my goal from staying abstinent to living the Steps did I know freedom from the obsession with food.

I am powerless over my abstinence. The moment I gave up my fight for it was the moment when God stepped in and took over my food addiction. Freedom was mine, and I know it can be yours too!

— *Bridgeport, Ohio USA*

Getting Back Up

Abstinence was not something that came easily to me. I still struggle some days, even after being in program eight years. I feel like abstinence was not an overnight, light-bulb moment. It occurred one baby step at a time. I managed to achieve the food plan that keeps me abstinent today only by not giving up.

I tried for years to do the all-or-nothing method, and that never worked. I kept coming back to meetings, though, and listening to members who had years of recovery. I took their suggestions one at a time, and when I saw it was working, I was ready to try another idea. I give a lot of credit to those who've gone before me and to my sponsor, who has nudged me in the right direction.

I don't immediately turn to the food. I use the tools: write, make a phone call, go to a meeting. They usually get me to the next day. This program is one day at a time.

I've managed to maintain a weight loss of 105 pounds (47 kg), and I can't imagine what my life would be today without this program. My favorite saying I live by is, "Failure is not falling down; it happens when you don't get back up again." I have to get back up, or my disease wins.

— *Baltimore, Maryland USA*

Coming Clean

After almost seven years in OA, I was in denial about working a "clean" recovery program. At first my weighing and measuring were never sloppy, but eventually I ignored cups and scales, thinking I could "eye-ball" the right amounts. Eating out became an excuse to overeat, bend rules, and ignore others. This gradual plunge into nonabstinence felt like quicksand. I thought I could get myself back on track.

I shuddered when the meeting leader asked for a moment of silence to pray for those suffering from compulsive eating in and out of the rooms. I thought, "That's me. I'm still hurting from this stinking disease that snuck up and grabbed me because I wouldn't face it." Oh, I used OA tools: meetings, calls to my sponsor, the Steps, sponsoring, service at meeting and intergroup levels, literature—all to convince myself and others I was working it.

Sometimes that inner voice urged me to come clean and tell my sponsor I had been lying about my food. I almost never weighed and measured it. I looked at some of my lowest-weight pictures to see the difference between my weight then and now. I tried to delude myself into believing my food was still abstinent despite my behavior. I understood the phrase "half-measures avail us nothing" (*Alcoholics Anonymous,* 4th ed., p. 59).

The last month I prayed for strength and courage to come clean with my food. God answered. A friend who had left the rooms years ago donated a box of OA literature. I had every book except the one on relapse, and I could relate to many of the stories. A few weeks later, my sponsor was leading my regular Saturday morning meeting. She passed out literature quotes and asked members to share, saying HP often gives us what we need in such a random process. I remember thinking, "Yeah, right! Miracles used to happen in the early days too." My snippet read, "Denial of the truth leads to destruction. Only an honest admission to ourselves of the reality of our condition can save us from our destructive eating" (*The Twelve Steps and Twelve Traditions of Overeaters Anonymous,* p. 6). "Oh, my God! It's a set up," I thought.

I mumbled a few words on the topic, not knowing what honest sharing to say. All day I went over what had happened. If this wasn't a sign, I didn't know what was. The next day I left on my sponsor's answering machine a message that seemed like a blessing because now she could call to let me go. I was so relieved, ashamed, and humiliated when she called; it didn't matter anymore. She guided me with love in doing the next right thing day by day. I met with my sponsor to talk about what had happened and to go over Step One after "coming clean."

She shared that a recent TV program had reminded her of my situation. A character on the show was trapped under a car in the middle of a desert. Death from lack of food or water would follow if the person didn't escape. Despite the extreme pain, it became necessary for survival and freedom for the character to break an arm. Denying my "eating" kept me trapped. Becoming honest was painful and humiliating. I want to live, so I had to come clean. I've been abstinent for almost two months, with my HP's help. Each day is easier, but I know none of us has this thing "licked." My disease is waiting and watching, but I cannot live in denial if I want any chance of maintaining abstinence. It feels so much better to have clean food.

— *Anonymous*

No More Traffic Cop

When I came to OA, I had a hard time getting abstinent. I had a loud inner critic whom my therapist named my "traffic cop." This male authoritarian figure embodied the abuse I had received; he controlled my self-esteem and body image.

When I looked in the mirror, I could not be objective about what I saw. I could only see the monster inside: the isolated, ashamed addict. I skewed my perception of my appearance so much that I was convinced I was the biggest person on my college campus (an absurd supposition). I thought all the skinny, tan girls were judging and criticizing me.

As a compulsive exerciser with bulimic tendencies and the body image of an anorexic, I came to OA to stop eating compulsively, to accept my body as it was, and to stop self-hating and trying to diet and binge myself into another shape. I wanted to be normal, but I soon learned normal wasn't an option for me. I had appropriated the insults and abuse I received from my partners over the years, and the traffic cop in my head made sure they still had power over me.

My therapist drew an image of the traffic cop and asked what I would like to say to him. I began crying. "It's not fair," I said, "that I try so hard every day to be a good person. I have done everything I can to live a right life. I'm doing everything I can to recover, to move on, but you're always there, keeping me from living my life. I don't want you anymore. You have no business being in my life."

That wasn't the last I heard of the traffic cop or the voices of my abusers, and I didn't magically adore my body after that. But recognizing I didn't want that voice to be part of my life made room for the voice of Higher Power. Slowly I began to look in the mirror and see not the distorted image of what I thought I was but myself as I was—an embodiment of the creative powers of the universe and a reflection of Higher Power.

I had a hard time with Step Two until I realized those voices of abuse kept me from coming to believe. If I look at myself with nonjudgmental eyes, I know I'm part of something greater—this Fellowship, the elements, the earth, the universe. The traffic cop is isolating, but OA brings me back to life again.

— Rohnert Park, California USA

The Moment it Clicked

I attended my first meeting on March 1, 1976. I was desperate. Over many years, I had lost a total of 85 pounds (39 kg) but had recently gained 27 pounds (12 kg)—while on a diet!

That night I heard the only requirement for membership is a desire to stop eating compulsively. To be truthful, I didn't have the requirement for membership. I only wanted to be thin. I had accepted I was meant to be miserable and afraid and couldn't do all the things that "normal" people seemed to do so easily and confidently. I didn't recognize my emotional and spiritual illness at the time, but I knew I needed help with my physical disease.

> *Soon, God willing, I will be abstinent sixteen years. Every day is a miracle.*

After eighteen months, even I saw that food plans worked in isolation in OA were no more effective than those I tried on my own. The people at my meeting said, "Stick with the winners." I noticed the winners were those who considered abstinence the most important thing in their lives and who worked the Steps.

Finally, on November 13, 1977, I called a sponsor and said I was willing to do whatever I had to do. "Whatever" began with a commitment to follow my food plan, no matter what. This commitment forced me to use the tools and the Steps in order to stay abstinent. The tools always got me back on the beam and in a place where I could work a Step. Through the Twelve Steps, my Higher Power worked a miracle—a total rearrangement of thoughts and motives such as the doctor describes in the Big Book. It did not happen quickly. I put many hours into meetings, retreats, and service, but the miracle did begin to take place. For this compulsive overeater, it couldn't have without abstinence from overeating first.

Since then, OA, my abstinence, and my food plan have all changed. I am not the same person I was, yet the framework of OA—the meetings, the Steps, the tools, prayer, and meditation—is still what I use to live this life I've been given. And abstaining from compulsive overeating still comes first for me.

I don't know what happened on November 13, 1977. It's best described as an awesome "click," as if a light had come on. My belief system had changed, and I chose to follow it. That first commitment to my food plan not only taught me how to make and keep other commitments, but it also gave me the gift of time—time to work the Steps without all the hopelessness, self-hate, and fear of pre-OA life. Soon, God willing, I will be abstinent sixteen years.

Every day is a miracle.

— Boulder, Colorado USA

Living in the Solution

Compulsive overeating had completely consumed me by the time I found my way into Overeaters Anonymous. My sole purpose in life was to eat, and at the same time, desperately seek a way to control my weight.

"Why can't I close the refrigerator door?" I'd wonder, tears pouring down my puffy face as I was eating nonstop from the top shelf to the bottom. I wanted to know why, on Saturday nights, when friends were out having fun, I was sitting at home in front of the television eating with both hands, at warp speed. And what sent me back for second, third, and fourth helpings when I wanted to stop at one?

> *It wasn't until I found Overeaters Anonymous that my insane behavior, thoughts, and feelings began to make sense.*

When not actively binge-eating, I was dieting, fasting, or visiting one more doctor, nutritionist, or acupuncturist. I hoped they'd show me the way out of the food, the fat, and my incessant mental and emotional turmoil.

It wasn't until I found Overeaters Anonymous that my insane behavior, thoughts, and feelings began to make sense. That first meeting nearly ten years ago showed me I wasn't alone. There were lots of others just like me who'd lost the power of choice when it came to food.

The men and women in these meetings knew my pain firsthand—they'd lived it. They offered me a road map that led me out of the problem and into the life-giving solution.

"Find a sponsor and a food plan you can follow," they suggested. "Make a commitment to a planned way of eating. Go regularly to meetings. Read the Big Book, *The Twelve Steps of Overeaters Anonymous*, and plenty of other OA literature. Reach out to others through the telephone. Above all, wholeheartedly work the Twelve Steps."

I couldn't imagine that recovery could hurt more than the torment of compulsive overeating, so I tried it. In the past decade, I've experienced major ups and downs—job changes, deaths, relocations, heartache, and joy—in short, life. But regardless of my degree of discomfort or elation, I've stayed clear of that first bite. I've followed the road map of recovery to the best of my ability, one day at a time. And I've found that living in the solution is the best way to go, under all conditions. Following this map has led me beyond my most heartfelt dreams: I'm healthy, happily married, and at peace with myself and the world around me most of the time. I've just written and published my first book. The love of friends surrounds me. I look forward to the future with an expectation of good. Traveling this road of recovery has shown me that there is a Higher Power—and this power is actively involved in every area of my life.

Positive things happen when I follow our program's directions, keep my feet firmly on the path of God's will, and walk with my head held high into the best that's yet to be.

— *Corona del Mar, California USA*

Trust to the Test

My ability to stay abstinent is being severely put to the test. My elderly mother is declining physically and mentally, causing deep concern for my family and me.

There doesn't seem to be a workable solution to allow her to receive proper care and at the same time keep her happy. To her, nothing is right; she sees only the negative.

In praying about the situation I realized that I, too, could easily start seeing only the negative. The more I prayed, the more I realized I needed to turn this problem over to my Higher Power. But I'm being asked to trust God in a way that scares me. I

> *In trying to trust God, I found some old, painful memories rising to the surface.*

want to control what happens to me and those I care about. But I can't do it in this situation.

In trying to trust God, I found some old, painful memories rising to the surface. My feelings were telling me to eat, that somehow I'd feel better. Instead I chose to talk my feelings out with someone I knew would listen without giving me a lot of advice. This made it easier to stay abstinent.

For me there is no solution, no love, no relief to be found in food. It's never made a bad situation better, only worse, because I only despise myself more for having overeaten.

Every day that I'm abstinent gives me the courage to trust God to get me through one more day. Instead of sleepless nights and worry-filled days, I'm finding serenity. I do what I can for my mother. I've forgiven her for the pain she caused me—and forgiven myself for the pain I've caused her.

I share with other family members how I'm coping with this difficult situation, how using the Twelve Steps of OA is deepening my trust in God. I see them struggle with their own distress over mom and pray for them, but I know I can't take their hurt away. Neither can I control what happens to them, make them stop eating compulsively, or make them work the Twelve Steps. They may need this program as much as I do, yet they must decide that for themselves.

But I can find peace with my lack of control. God loves them as much as me. If they should hit bottom, God will be there to help them, too.

As for me, my only choice today is to trust God—and stay abstinent.

— *Ellisville, Missouri USA*

Back in the Game

I recently received a phone call informing me that a friend was extremely ill and might not live much longer. This really shook me up because I love my friend very much but had never told him so and, in fact, hadn't talked to him in months.

When I received this news I was practicing my food addiction and initially I ate over it, although I wish I could say I didn't. But then something happened. My Higher Power wouldn't let me isolate myself any longer.

Feeling desperate, I wrote and mailed a letter expressing my love to my friend, something I've wanted to do for a long time. I made direct amends for isolating myself and neglecting our relationship. At the time I didn't know whether he'd still be alive to receive my letter, but I was able to leave this in the hands of my Higher Power.

At that moment, I was given the gift of abstinence. Suddenly I knew that my active disease is what had kept me from really being there in our relationship, and I was finally entirely ready to have God remove this defect of character.

Incidentally my friend did receive my letter. He wrote back, and I went to see him. I cherish the memory of that visit.

I've decided that no matter what, I'm going to choose relationships over food. I've been to two parties since then, and I've been able to remain abstinent, focusing on the people rather than the food.

One of the parties was with some of my spouse's business associates. Although I hardly knew anyone, I still had a good time. Instead of my usual fear, I went to the party with the thought that "these are people I might like to get to know." But there was a time when the very idea of socializing would have been just too scary.

I have several more social gatherings to attend, and I'm praying that God will help me continue to be there for the people instead of the food.

I'm working on my relationship with my spouse as well. It's really scary. But nothing is as scary as the thought that I might again practice my disease, neglect my relationships, but this time, not have a second chance.

— *Austin, Texas USA*

Taking My Medicine

My obsession with food began in the high chair. I have vague memories of my mother feeding me as she and my father argued. As the dispute grew more and more heated, and my mother more nervous, she'd start feeding me faster and faster. The message I received from this was that food was the way to deal with everything.

> *The first time around in OA, abstinence had come so gently and easily. This time it was a struggle.*

The marriage dissolved a short time later. Unfortunately my compulsion didn't.

I found my way to OA in 1988 after a bout with cancer. The program helped me get my life together and gave me a way to deal with the fear of recurrence by teaching me to live one day at a time. I got abstinent at my first meeting, and in four months I reached goal weight. I felt wonderful.

In retrospect, I see that I'd concentrated on the numbers. I counted every calorie, and weighed and measured myself instead of the food. I used all the tools of recovery but never worked the Steps beyond the third. I needed to get back into life and thought being slim would assist the process.

Being thin, however, doesn't necessarily mean being well. Inside I was the same even though my appearance had changed. I found a job after being unemployed for more than a year. Claiming fatigue I stopped going to meetings. Five months later I relapsed, beginning a two-year physical, emotional, and spiritual descent into hell. I denied to myself that I looked any different, even as I was slowly putting all the weight back on, and more.

Twice during that time I attempted to return to the program. Both times I wasn't ready or willing and after a couple of weeks I gave up.

In May of 1991 I hit bottom. I returned to OA, making a commitment to attend a meeting a day for as long as it would take to get abstinent. There was nowhere else to go. It was "do it or die"—literally.

The first week back in OA was exciting, and the feeling of not being out of control was new and liberating. Now that I wasn't eating constantly, my poor stomach could let me know when I was truly hungry. But I was still eating sugar, telling myself I needed to get off it "slowly." After a week of meetings, I had to be honest; it was time to get clean and sober. For me that meant no sugar at all.

The second and third weeks were difficult. I was abstinent but sick from the withdrawal, tense, angry, nauseated. My sleep was disturbed, and I was tired.

The first time around in OA, abstinence had come so gently and easily. This time it was a struggle. Those two weeks made a definite impression on me. I'd suffered for this abstinence. It wouldn't be so casually thrown away again.

I'd go to meetings feeling ill and wanting to leave, but by meeting's end, the symptoms would stop. I began to understand that meetings truly were my medicine.

After three weeks of this I thought I was "all set," and I cut down to one meeting a week. I soon became aware that my abstinence was in jeopardy, and went back to attending a meeting a day, eventually settling on a three-meetings-a-week schedule.

Today is my seventieth day of abstinence. I'm a sponsor for the first time, and I'm receiving so much more from my sponsee than I could ever give. I'm losing weight very slowly and I'm content with that. I no longer own a scale. As I grow stronger and saner each day, the weight will come off.

This time I'm in the program for keeps. I'm so very grateful to be a recovering compulsive overeater.

— *Fall River, Massachusetts USA*

The Reprieve

I'm a rock-bottom, in-the-gutter type of compulsive eater, now abstinent and recovering by the grace of God. Whenever I speak at a meeting, my sponsor always reminds me beforehand to tell my "I almost died" story. It's important for me to keep the memory green, and also vital to let the people listening to me know exactly how bad things can get.

I won't go into the gory details here. Suffice it to say that I had no less than five life-threatening physical problems when I came back into OA after my relapse, all of which were directly related to compulsive overeating and purging.

When I returned to OA, it took me a while to get abstinent. The sixth attempt was the one that produced lasting abstinence. I think it happened not because I was finally ready and willing at that point, but because the sixth withdrawal nearly finished me off. When I stopped vomiting, fainting, seeing and hearing hallucinations, and feeling suicidally depressed, I had learned one important thing: If I overeat again, it might kill me. I couldn't afford to risk even a slip—it might trigger a fatal relapse.

My first time around in OA, I was one of those people who refused to follow a food plan. At the age of twenty-two, and in a very early stage of my compulsive eating, I didn't need to. But my disease progressed rapidly over the last few years. There are foods which I could eat moderately my first time in OA which I cannot consume safely now. I have to watch my food-related activities and emotions very carefully. I can't afford the occasional slips I had when I was in OA the first time. I need to maintain consistent abstinence in order to survive.

I no longer feel a need to rebel against food planning. Every evening after dinner, I write down what I plan to eat the next day and call it in to my sponsor. I carry it around on a little 3x5 inch (8x13 cm) card. If something isn't on the plan, I don't eat it. I have learned from painful experience that I cannot make moderate choices about food when I am hungry. I plan my food when I have a full stomach, and I don't deviate from that plan.

I have been cleanly abstinent for 109 glorious days as I write this article. I have lost 51 pounds (23 kg) and my physical health is much improved through not carrying that extra weight. My health is excellent. All five life-threatening conditions reversed themselves within the first two months of abstinence. My emotional condition is much better, too. Instead of being depressed, exhausted, and cynical, I feel joyful, energetic, and full of hope for the future.

As I continue to abstain, work the Steps, and use the tools of recovery, I realize how badly off I was before I returned to OA. My husband sometimes comments that he is living with a different person. It's a wonder our marriage survived the progression of my illness; I was a bitter, sick, unhappy person for several years.

I'm not trying to suggest that everything is now perfect. My health has not yet completely returned, I occasionally fall prey to exhaustion, and my immune system is still not normal. Every cold or virus that's going around finds me and puts me through the wringer. But I no longer greet each day with a migraine and end it with heart palpitations, wondering whether I will survive another day or even if I want to survive. By the grace of God and the power of the OA program, I have been given the greatest gift of all: a daily reprieve from the deadly illness of compulsive eating. It is worth any amount of effort to maintain that.

— *Wilmington, Delaware USA*

It Works if You Work It

The disease of compulsive overeating is cunning, baffling, and powerful. It uses any means possible to rob us of our program and recovery, manipulating us into continuing to use excess food for survival. It keeps us in the bondage of food, fat, overeating, and self-obsession. The disease cuts us off from the world and closes the pathway to God.

Our recovery is contingent on the elimination of compulsive overeating from our lives so that we can reopen that pathway and keep it clear. It's only through abstinence that we can do that.

The Twelve Steps and Twelve Traditions of Overeaters Anonymous focuses on freedom from compulsive eating. I believe that this concept encourages us not only to eliminate behaviors such as bingeing, eating certain foods, or eating at certain times and places, but also to eliminate all those behaviors that tend to lead us into compulsive eating, and those that allow us to find comfort in food, be it excess or not.

To those of us who've come a long way emotionally, spiritually, and physically, but who still carry excess weight (of which I am one), I can only say that it's the continuous elimination of compulsive eating behaviors that leads to continued recovery from this disease.

As long as I'm overweight, I'm eating more food than my body needs, and if I'm eating more than I need, I'm overeating. Simple overeating leads to compulsive overeating—which can lead me right out of the program. And some who leave the program never find their way back.

I have to take my abstinence seriously. Everything else in my life must revolve around it. There's no other road to recovery for me but the one paved with abstinence, and there's no other guidance on that road but my spirituality. The two go hand in hand. I can't have one without the other.

If I remain overweight, then there are still some food choices and eating behaviors that I'm not turning over to God. It means I've not enriched my spiritual life enough to eliminate these things. I must continue to eliminate them if I want continued recovery. No matter where I am in recovery or how much I weigh, I must always be willing to turn over more than I think I need to, especially when it comes to food.

No, thinness doesn't mean wellness—but being overweight doesn't either. I believe I can be free of the compulsion and the fat. There's nothing to fear. God will take me there if I'm willing to give up the crutch of excess food. I have to get out of my own way and let God do the work.

— *Hickory, North Carolina USA*

Worthwhile Struggle

For me, the disease of compulsive overeating began with graze eating and occasional binges. Over the years it progressed to daily binges, midnight raids of the refrigerator, and all the humiliating behaviors that came with trying to satisfy my craving for more—taking food back out of the trash can; gorging myself at salad bars, banquets, and potlucks; and eating with two hands, wishing I had three. But, of course, "more" was never enough.

The evening that I made an unconditional surrender to abstinence and to a Higher Power, I'd felt anything but faith. I was full of food, full of fear, and had only the tiniest hope that I could live free of excess food and correct the unmanageable life that my compulsive overeating had created.

> *God saw me through the food withdrawals, gave me the power to avoid my "first bite," and led me into a richly rewarding new life.*

During my bingeing days, there were times I could not shut the pantry or refrigerator door for fear of being separated from food. The thought of going from breakfast to lunch, lunch to dinner, and dinner to bedtime without eating in between seemed overwhelming.

Yet I knew I couldn't go on eating and living under the lashes of this progressive and fatal disease. I adopted a three-meal-a-day abstinence, staying away from second helpings, snacks, and binge foods. I asked God to help me keep this commitment under all conditions. I began the withdrawal process that taxed my body, mind, and emotions beyond anything I had ever experienced.

It is painfully clear to me why a return to the disease of compulsive overeating seems an attractive alternative to enduring the initial withdrawal symptoms. Newly abstinent, I recall crying when I'd finished my meals. I wanted more! I watched "normal" folks eat dessert with impunity; why couldn't I? And many nights I lay awake, food calling to me.

Sometimes, when the craving to eat was very strong, I'd take a shower, take a walk, or make a phone call. I knew that the only way out of the disease for me was to avoid the first bite, with God's help. I was, and still am, willing to go to any length to recover.

I often had to turn down the volume on the mental voice that said it was okay to have "just a little" food. I learned to reprogram my thinking through OA literature and meetings. My emotions during that time were strong and varied. Dealing with relationships, work, and daily living became a minute-by-minute challenge.

Why did I endure that anguish when I knew that food could temporarily straighten out my thoughts, feelings, and physical discomfort? Because I wanted to be mentally free, emotionally alive, and physically healthy. I had to believe that these withdrawal symptoms would not last. Hope and faith, if only a little, were my guiding lights.

It's been more than six years since I made my commitment to abstinence. God saw me through the food withdrawals, gave me the power to avoid my "first bite," and led me into a richly rewarding new life. It hasn't been a pain-free journey, yet the freedom I feel has been worth every effort. I could not then, nor can I now, make this journey alone. I need each and every one of you to walk with me.

— *Corona del Mar, California USA*

It's a Personal Choice

For several years I have wrestled with the question of whether alcohol could be a part of my plan of abstinence from compulsive overeating. I never thought of myself as an alcoholic. I didn't fit my image of an alcoholic; I didn't even like the word. Yes, you could say I abused alcohol, but that occasional abuse seemed like nothing when compared to my daily abuse of food.

Food was always my drug of choice. Destructive relationships came next. Alcohol was not even a close third. So I convinced myself that I could be abstinent and still drink occasionally. I could control it. And, for the most part, I did control it. I cut down substantially on my drinking, reserving it for special occasions.

But even after four years in OA, my abstinence from compulsive overeating never lasted for more than a few months at a time. While I may have thought I was able to handle alcohol, I knew I wasn't able to handle the aftereffects of drinking. I found that when I drink, abstinence from compulsive overeating and from destructive relationships seems much less important.

Can alcohol be a part of my abstinence? I think not. It's not worth the price of my abstinence. Nothing is.

— *Loudonville, New York USA*

Crucial Step

I had been in Overeaters Anonymous for almost three years and had lost 130 pounds (59 kg). My relationship with God was the most important part of my recovery. I truly believed that God was removing my obsession with food. Then it happened. Relapse. I started gaining a little weight and became consumed by the fear of regaining it all. I expressed this fear to many OA friends. While I will

I felt hopeless but I kept showing up at meetings several times a week.

always be grateful for their constant friendship during this trying time, I was unable to accept their help.

The problem was that I had stopped believing in Step Two, and was totally unwilling to practice Step Three. During the next three years I gained back all my weight plus a little extra. I felt hopeless but I kept showing up at meetings several times a week. Often I considered not going because I was afraid newcomers would look at me and wonder if the program worked. Even so, I continued to go to meetings because I knew that OA and its principles were my only hope for a better life.

But what was wrong?

Finally someone suggested that I do a spiritual inventory. The seed was planted.

For weeks I considered doing the inventory, but I didn't know how to begin. I summoned the courage to ask the person who'd suggested it if she would recommend some issues I might address. I firmly believe God had placed this precious person in my life.

I followed some of her suggestions and was amazed at the outpouring of conflicts that existed between me and Higher Power. When I gave away my spiritual inventory, I realized that I needed to reevaluate my concept of God and determine what God could and would do for me. Until I took this Step, I was unable to believe that a Power greater than myself would restore my abstinence.

It was hard for me to develop my own concept of God, but once I did, I was able to turn over the extra food, the food thoughts, and my fear of dying from compulsive overeating. I have been able to stay abstinent one day at a time for nine weeks. I now want to be abstinent more than I want to overeat. This is truly a miracle from my loving Higher Power, because I was almost certain I would never experience recovery again. But God can and will do for me what I am unable to do for myself as long as I believe God alone has the power.

— *Leavenworth, Kansas USA*

Abstinent and Smoke-Free

At the basis of my disease was an inability to accept myself the way I am—6 feet 1 inch (186 cm), left-handed, flat-chested, large-hipped. As the child of an alcoholic, I learned the art of self-loathing early in life. My adolescence was acutely painful; by the age of fifteen, food was my chief comfort and self-derision was my favorite pastime.

I'd always known I was a compulsive overeater. I was also aware that if I drank much at all, I would probably become an alcoholic. So I avoided booze, but I ate instead. I survived to mid-life on the yo-yo cycle of pills and diets, very often depressed.

> By working the OA program and with very definite help from my Higher Power who removed my desire for cigarettes—I was able to quit.

I began my recovery from compulsive overeating at the same time my alcoholic parent joined AA. I went to OA meetings because I wanted to contribute to the health of my family, not because I was motivated by self-love. During the first year, I continued to overeat (so for a long time I did not count that year as "recovery"), but I gave up my major addictions to destructive relationships and drugs. I got a sponsor and worked the Steps. I trained myself to eat only three meals a day and went to every OA meeting I could.

The second year, I found a very lanky sponsor and tried a food plan she suggested. I shrank to a weight even thinner than what I'd weighed when I was twelve; I felt like a child again. My menstrual cycle ceased for the next three years. I had no idea that anorexia was part of my disease. It was only through the loving confrontations and support of OA friends that I found the courage to let go of my rigidity concerning food.

My years in OA have been ones of personal growth; in them, I have come face-to-face with enormous amounts of fear. It seemed that behind each fear was another, an endless supply of terror that kept me clinging to anything that offered security.

My best friends were my cigarettes. It took me a long, long time to admit that smoking hampered my recovery by masking my feelings. I knew I was still "using" but I was terrified I'd gain weight if I quit. How could I, abstinent so long, quit smoking and risk losing control?

By working the OA program—and with very definite help from my Higher Power who removed my desire for cigarettes—I was able to quit. The miracle is that I only gained about 15 pounds (7 kg), which I've read is a typical weight gain experienced by people who quit smoking. At times my abstinence was a two on a scale of one-to-ten, but not once was I drawn to my old ally, sugar.

I can't minimize the experience of quitting smoking; it was awful, terrible at times. But the Twelve-Step program made it possible. Over and over I said to myself, "Nobody said this would be easy, but it is possible." I grieved my smokes. I cried for no reason. I suffered anxiety attacks. I went to lots of meetings.

In July of last year, I celebrated seven years of abstinence in OA, my fortieth birthday, and one year without cigarettes. I am very happy with myself. This is the reason: I accept myself today just as I am—forty years old, wrinkling, single, a size bigger, and not a bit richer. I love me. What a gift I have given myself. What miracles have come from just three little words—"Keep coming back."

— *Santa Cruz, California USA*

Footwork of Abstinence

When I first came into the OA program, I asked my HP for the gift of abstinence. I didn't receive it on a silver platter. Then I asked for the willingness to be abstinent, and I didn't receive that on a silver platter either. I had limited success and felt justified in saying, "I am leaving it up to my HP." I left the rooms and went into relapse.

> *All I have to remember is that abstinence is an action.*

When I came back, a member with more than 15 years of abstinence asked me if I was abstinent. I said, "I asked for willingness but am not quite in the mood yet." She reminded me that abstinence is an action, and mood has nothing to do with it. She was right about that. I have been abstinent for a couple of years now, and many times I am not in the mood. All I have to remember is that abstinence is an action. That is what the term "white-knuckle abstinence" means to me. It means being abstinent even when the world is falling apart; even when it is the only thing that goes right that day; even when your HP isn't answering your prayers, and you need comfort somewhere. Those are the days I work my program.

These days, I ask for the willingness to work the Steps and deal with the feelings and the issues. I pray for the willingness to do yet another mini-inventory and seek to make the amends that smooth out my life. I ask for the willingness to make the changes my HP asks for to have my defects removed. I don't ask for the willingness to be abstinent because that is the commitment I made to my HP.

What do I get instead of the temporary comfort of excess food when I commit to abstinence as my footwork? I get the resentments, anger, and obsession with food out of my life. That is the gift my HP gives me for doing the footwork of abstinence and working the Steps.

— *Sharpsburg, Georgia USA*

CHAPTER FOUR

Abstinence Is a Priority

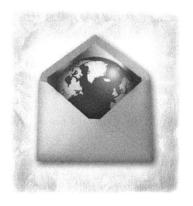

Stick Around

In the past, dieting was my game, and making promises to myself. I would promise never to weigh more than 25 pounds (11 kg) over my weight at the time. At 175 pounds (80 kg), I swore I would never reach 200 pounds (91 kg). If I did, that would be it! I'd have to do something: at least cut back on my food consumption, or even another diet might be the answer. This went on for 25 pounds (11 kg) at a time until I reached 275 pounds (125 kg). I just could not stop eating. If I did, it was not for long. Yes, diets were successful. Not that successful, though. I would just start to eat again, putting lost weight back on and adding a few more pounds.

I was in the grip of something beyond my control, but I didn't know what. One thing for sure, I was not eating to live. I was living to eat, a dangerous game. None of the solutions I tried seemed to work over the long haul. I was good for the sprint, not the marathon.

Hearing about Overeaters Anonymous in my hometown caught my attention. Maybe this program would be an answer for me. At first, what kept me coming back was hearing a recovering compulsive overeater share he no longer found it necessary to consume large quantities of food at a sitting. That is what I was doing. He had lost a considerable amount of weight and was keeping the weight off. That's what I wanted!

I discovered in OA I was a compulsive overeater and was afflicted by an illness with a physical symptom, an emotional problem with a spiritual solution. It was not a moral issue or social problem. It was an illness. I learned I had been eating gross amounts of food to satisfy an emotional hunger and fill a spiritual void—an impossible feat. Believe me, I tried.

I further learned abstinence must become the most important thing in my life. At the time, abstinence was refraining from compulsive overeating. More learning and experiences came along the way. Abstinence now encompasses far more.

Abstinence is a gift from God given to me at birth. I had either abused, misused, or did not use the gift. OA has guided me. The Fellowship has supported me. God has overseen my journey. All I had to be was willing to go to every length to keep abstinence first.

More than thirty-two years later, abstinence remains most important in my life. Maintaining a weight loss of about 110 pounds (50 kg) proves physical recovery is attainable. I still have ongoing work one day at a time. Daily prayer work, daily footwork, and continued willingness contribute to a healthier life. I don't just keep coming back; I just stick around. By doing so, I won't be so round again.

— *Windsor, Colorado USA*

No Matter What

I don't have another option other than abstinence. The only other way I know to lose weight is to go on a diet. But diets end, and then what? Plus, there is the last meal or binge one eats before a diet begins. So I abstain to lose weight, maintain my weight loss, avail myself of the many promises mentioned in the Big Book, and live a sane and satisfying life.

My abstinence is writing down what I eat every day, no matter what: healthy food, unhealthy food, moderate portions, gigantic amounts, candy or carrots, I write it down!

No matter what I'm feeling or how busy I am, I write down my food. No matter if I change my mind and eat something else, I write it down or cross it out and rewrite it. No matter what, no matter what, no matter what, I write down what I eat.

It took me over five years to define and commit to this abstinence. It began as the result of my sponsor asking me what I was willing to do, no matter what. To answer this simple question, I had to go through trial and error to simplify the elaborate plans that first came to mind.

Then I created another problem. I compared myself to other OA members. My abstinence wasn't like what others did, or so I thought. I hadn't been successful when trying to eat only three meals a day (I ate four), and I couldn't imagine giving up sugar or flour. But remember, my sponsor asked me what I was willing to do, not what I thought I should do.

So, you may ask, from what do I abstain? I wondered that myself. What a relief when another OA member gave me the answer: I abstain from dishonesty. And yes, some foods I don't eat. I looked back and was able to identify three foods I used to binge on but haven't eaten since I came to OA. I've added a few more to the list over the years, but my willingness to write down what I eat means more to me than what foods I eat or don't eat.

One day at a time, I abstain, and that's been going on for about nineteen years.

— *Burbank, California USA*

Bye-Bye, Seconds

I have been an OA member for over fifteen years. God blessed me with the gift of abstinence at the beginning of my wonderful journey in OA. Over the years, with God doing for me what I can't do for myself, I've almost always had a comfortable abstinence. Although I never ate between meals or binged, sugar became an issue at times, and I made poor food choices.

Gradually, I began to gain weight. Thanks to a dear sponsee who chose the topic of hope when she led our meeting, I realized I had become comfortable being overweight and had no hope that I could ever lose weight. That night God, through this blessed messenger, gave me hope again, along with true freedom from compulsive eating and the willingness to give up desserts and second helpings one day at a time.

I can't begin to tell you how much better I feel physically, emotionally, and spiritually. I've experienced a significant weight loss, but more important, abstinence is again the most important thing in my life without exception. God is back to being number one in my life, right where he belongs.

It pays to attend OA meetings regularly. You never know what you might hear that can change your life, or what you might say that could change someone else's.

Keep coming back. It works!

— *Palms, California USA*

Taking Action

How elusive is abstinence! It darts in and out, scaring the socks off us!

Some people can live with it, but I couldn't until I got a food plan—my very own, designed specifically for my needs—and until working the Steps taught me how to live with abstinence.

Other changes in my life have come from working the Steps, and I have my sponsor to thank for this. Nancy didn't start out as my sponsor. I never called her or asked her for help. (I had telephone phobia, you understand. I knew how to isolate myself.) She was just a friend in program working her Twelfth Step who called me one day and asked, "How've you been?" And then she meddled, telling me, "You know, you're never going to get anywhere until you do your Fourth Step."

Oh, the Fourth Step. I had abstained from that as well as the food. I realized I had to do it, so I asked Nancy if I could read it to her. In my Fifth Step, she lived through my long, woeful accounts of who'd done me wrong and where I was to blame, and all the ugliness in my life reared its head. Character defects, I believe they're called. I had yet to learn about those.

Nancy was so gracious. Her eyes only glazed over once while I read. When I finished, she hugged me and told me I was okay. She understood. She knew what I was talking about.

I practice other abstinences as well. I now abstain from jealousy, which used to be my big thing. I'm learning to walk away from pride and let it shrivel up and die! I abstain from worrying, and I'm learning to trust that others can take care of themselves. I refrain from nagging and trying to control other people—I used to major in those. Now I just take one day at a time and live and let live. I wonder where I got that—program, perhaps?

I also stay away from slippery people, places, and things, which for me are drive-throughs, church dinners, and certain family celebrations; yet I've realized abstinence goes deeper than our behavior in a kitchen or at a restaurant. It touches every area of our lives. Abstinence requires a life plan, not simply a food plan. That's why we have the Twelve Steps. That's why we have a program.

We will never be abstinent from compulsive overeating as long as we talk about it. We will forever sit on the sidelines and long for what others have, feeling flawed and inadequate ourselves. Abstinence is an action. To have what they have, we have to be willing. We have to reach out. We have to accept. We have to find out and do what they did. And if we see someone drowning in our midst, too overwhelmed by life to utter the word "help," we can throw out the lifeline.

Does abstinence come overnight? For some, yes; but for many of us, gaining it is a process. Within the past two years, my mother has died, my father-in-law has had cancer, my brother-in-law has become terminally ill, and we've moved twice. I would have kicked against all this at one time. Now I accept it. I'm taking it one day at a time, one Step at a time. I'm finding serenity and—amazingly enough—the ability to refrain from compulsive overeating. Nothing has happened overnight, but it has happened. The key is to keep coming back. It works if you work it. Some of us have to work it a long time. Then one day, as if by magic, something clicks, and we've made it.

We may find we don't have perfect abstinence, but we learn from our humanness and we go on. We learn to think, to act on life rather than react to it, to accept what we can't do anything about, and to change what we can. We can only change our actions, our thought processes, and our patterns of interacting.

Abstinence is my hiding place. Where I once turned to food, I now turn to this safe haven where I take care of myself and entrust my family to the God of my understanding. That's not a bad place to be.

Begin this process by loving yourself. Work the Steps with the help of God and a sponsor. You can find abstinence, joy, and peace. That is OA's gift. Receive it! You deserve to be abstinent.

— *Ocean City, Maryland USA*

A Pivotal Decision

I am celebrating nine years of abstinence. For someone who couldn't stay on a diet for longer than three days, that's a miracle—a miracle made possible by OA.

Nine years ago I'd been in OA for four years and had seldom had more than a few days of abstinence. I looked at those who had been abstinent for years and concluded they must not have the same disease.

In those four years I couldn't make much headway with the Steps because I didn't have a firm foundation of Step One on which to build my recovery. Driven by fear, desperation, and borrowed hope, however, I did learn to use the tools. I got over my fear of making calls, even to those with long-term abstinence. I performed service by setting up chairs and laying out literature at meetings. I formed small relapse recovery groups in my home. I wrote. I meditated. I read program literature.

So I made the commitment to identify the first compulsive bite and call someone before taking it.

Since childhood, fear had led me to a strict self-reliance. Only from the agony of compulsive overeating was I propelled to reach out to others for help. After four years in OA I had enough despair and enough hope to surrender completely. I had admitted powerlessness before but not that my life was totally unmanageable. After a week of abstinence I wrote a Fourth-Step inventory and read it to a friend who had six years of abstinence.

I wavered back and forth on the way home. If I wanted what my friend had—long-term abstinence, clarity, self-respect, recovery—I had to commit 100 percent to abstinence. But what about the "freedom" of eating what and when I wanted? I had a choice: discipline and recovery or "freedom" and sickness. My Higher Power intervened. I made the decision for abstinence.

But how? After four years of trying and failing, what could I do differently? How could I be sure I would never again, one day at a time, slip back into compulsive overeating? Many times I'd read the OA pamphlet *Before You Take That First Compulsive Bite, Remember* . . . and agreed with it completely. Yet time and time again I ended up back in the food. Why? Because I didn't always know what the first compulsive bite was. Only occasionally did I dive right into a binge; usually I slid there.

So I made the commitment to identify the first compulsive bite and call someone before taking it. Nine years of abstinence began with a single meal. I am no nearer to overeating today than I was nine years ago, and no further either—I'm still just one bite away.

Nine years of practice, commitment, and working the Steps have kept me from taking that bite. I turned my food over to a sponsor for the first few years. I couldn't avoid all the binge foods as I'd binged on practically everything, but I did avoid my main ones. I could then fully work the Steps, confident that the pain, fear, anger, and joy would not send me back to food. I got honest and clear about what I was eating. I could then learn to be honest about everything else.

A lot has changed in nine years. I eat all kinds of foods now with no cravings, obsession, or compulsion to overeat—I don't plan my meals in advance or commit them to someone unless I'm under great stress and find it comforting to do so. One thing has not changed, however. Whether I'm eating at home, a picnic, a buffet, a restaurant, or a friend's house, I always make the decision as to what the first compulsive bite would be, and commit to make a call before taking it.

My life is wonderful today. I am engaged to be married. I am about to go back to school. The promises have come true for me. It all began with abstinence and my decision to recognize and call before that first compulsive bite nine years ago.

— *Glorieta, New Mexico USA*

The Abstinence Advantage

Abstinence is the most important thing in my life today without exception. It hasn't always been. I've maintained a 65-pound (29-kg) weight loss since coming to OA three and a half years ago, in spite of many ups and downs with abstinence. Recently I was once again humbled by my addiction to food, especially sweets. I now know that no matter what does—or doesn't—happen, today will be a success if I remain abstinent. I can say that because I realize more than ever that only when I am abstinent and free from my overwhelming obsession with food am I able to put other things in my life in perspective. When my focus is on food, everything else is out of focus. I used to cringe when I heard people say that abstinence was the most important thing in their lives. More important than God? I thought that was blasphemy. Now I realize that unless I am abstinent, I can't put God first. When I'm overeating, food becomes my god. I worship it and trust it to make things better. When I am abstinent, I put my trust in God and I'm free to live the rich, full life God has in mind for me.

A major symptom or characteristic of my disease is recurring episodes of insanity.

Sometimes, however, I still forget why it is so important for me to abstain from sweets and from overeating. I've spent the last three and a half years since coming into OA experimenting with various eating plans in an effort to define my own personal abstinence. I've proven over and over, beyond a shadow of a doubt, that when I eat sweets my obsession with food returns and my compulsion takes over my whole life. Even though I know I can be free from the misery that accompanies my obsession simply by abstaining, I still find myself rationalizing and trying to justify eating "just this one sweet thing." Why? Because at least where food is concerned, I'm not sane.

A major symptom or characteristic of my disease is recurring episodes of insanity. During these attacks I forget the pain and misery of compulsive overeating and lose sight of the reasons for abstinence. Abstinence suddenly seems silly, or impossible, or overrated! I think, "What's the big deal about abstinence?" Later, of course, after I've given in to the urge to overeat, my sanity returns, and I realize the price I have paid for once again having given in to my disease.

Knowing that I am subject to insanity regarding food, I am learning to talk myself through these situations. I tell myself: "Right now abstinence doesn't seem very important, but that's because of the insanity. I have temporarily forgotten I am a compulsive overeater and have lost sight of the reality of my disease."

But somewhere inside me a tiny, soft-spoken voice (the sane part of me) assures me that remaining abstinent really is the most important thing I can do today. Maybe I don't feel like abstinence is very important at that moment, but it is essential that I remember that feelings cannot always be trusted. I must listen to the little voice of sanity, however weak it may be. I must trust that, in time, the insanity will pass, and I will once again remember why abstinence is so vital.

Now that I'm more aware of the nature of my insanity, perhaps I can learn to recognize the early warning signs before the episodes become full-blown. Maybe I can better recognize the distorted thinking that accompanies these attacks. And maybe it will become easier for me to listen to the quiet voice inside of me. Perhaps the voice will become stronger each time I listen to it.

This disease will be with me all my life and I presume I will always be subject to these recurring episodes of insanity. But there is a method of treatment. The Big Book tells me the good news: There is a solution. There is a way of living which allows me to have a daily reprieve from my illness, as long as I work the Steps and am willing to do whatever it takes to have recovery.

— *Sylacauga, Alabama USA*

Abstinence—It's Not a Numbers Game

Last night during pitch time I said my piece. But I left the meeting wondering if what I said was what I meant to say. My heart was going out to newcomers and others who have not quite been able to "let go and let God" help them with their abstinence.

Because many OA members in my area are blessed with great gifts of long-standing abstinence, our meetings are often abstinence-oriented. This is a wonderful thing for us, and exactly what I need.

But I have noticed that some of our newcomers and a few of our diligent but nonabstinent members are either dropping out or fighting their reluctance to attend meetings. Because they are not currently abstinent, they are feeling "less than" others.

OA is not a diet club, but it's not an abstinence-seniority club either. OA is a program that uses the Twelve Steps to help compulsive overeaters find peace, health, and recovery from their food obsession. The first day of abstinence for a newcomer is just as important as day 2,347 for a longtimer.

Often I begin my pitch with, "Hi! I'm C.W, and I'm a compulsive overeater, and this is my _____ day/month/year of abstinence." For me, my abstinence is something to celebrate. But, thinking back, perhaps I've been a little smug. As I have remained abstinent through the generosity of my HP, I have gained more compassion for those still compulsively overeating. I have noticed smiles freeze on faces and eyes show despair every time a member proclaims his or her length of abstinence.

So, after much deliberation, I've decided to change my little introduction. From now on I'll say, "Hi, I'm C.W., and I'm a compulsive overeater, and thanks to my HP, *today* I am abstinent." When they pass around the sheet that lists abstinence birthdays, I won't add my name.

Still, I wonder about what I said last night. I do have a tendency to sound preachy; I'd like to fix everyone and everything—anything to distract me from my problems. Although I have definite opinions about the competition that can result when comparing one member's length of abstinence to another's, I have an even stronger conviction about the concept of abstinence. Before my commitment to abstinence in OA, I allowed greed, self-centeredness, jealousy, and envy to consume me. I was miserable, and I made sure that those closest to me knew it. On the other hand, in my public life I was cheerful and witty, and I would often go out of my way for those who would give me approval or attention. I was at the mercy of my disease for thirty-two years; I don't want to go back.

Abstinence is absolutely essential to peace and sanity. It is more important than anything to me—more than my religious beliefs and more than my love for my husband, children, and family. And they are all worth going to any length for! You see, if I am not abstinent, I cannot appreciate or participate in those wonders. Abstinent for today, I see with new eyes a world I occupied all my life but never saw: a child's struggles, a husband's disappointment, a beautiful landscape. Abstinent for today, I am willing to go to a movie or a play without the promise that I'll be taken out for a huge dinner also. Abstinent for today, I find that my children are for loving, hugging, fussing over, and holding hands with: not for showering with the tons of sugared treats I bought for them but ate by myself instead.

So, if you were at that meeting and I left you a little confused, I apologize. In the future you won't find me listing my abstinence in number of days. But don't let that fool you—it's still the most important thing in my life.

— *Aloha, Oregon USA*

Handle With Care

I finally made it—thirty days of abstinence!

I have had several weeks of abstinence a number of times, but I usually broke it about the twenty-fifth or twenty-sixth day. I always sabotaged myself in some way as I neared the "magical" thirty-day mark. Now that that day has come and gone, I realize there is nothing magical about thirty days per se; but there is something miraculous about every day of abstinence.

As I neared the thirty-day mark this most recent time, I saw how poorly I had been treating my very fragile abstinence. I was handling it carelessly, playing with it, almost daring myself to break it. This was most apparent to me during the celebration of a recent holiday.

As part of my personal plan, I chose to refrain from the traditional binge foods that had always represented joy and celebration, and replaced them with good, wholesome foods that my entire family could enjoy. To establish a festive feeling, I prepared the table with the best of everything—fancy place mats, our best china, crystal goblets (not used since our wedding), and a crystal candle holder at each setting.

The only thing "out of place," so to speak, was a cheaper, smaller glass goblet that I set before my six-year-old daughter. I felt I couldn't quite trust her to handle a large crystal goblet. She cried when she saw that she had a different glass, until she noticed that it, too, was fancy and delicate.

As she handled the smaller goblet, I felt my heart leap into my throat several times. She treated it so roughly, pretending to be toasting with everyone, hitting the glass against every available surface, and setting it down a bit too hard after every gulp.

Suddenly, I saw myself in her. I had been handling my abstinence roughly also. As I'd seen the thirty-day mark approach, I was so sure I would break my abstinence again that I toyed with it. I let myself taste things that I had no business tasting. I wasn't caring for my abstinence lovingly or carefully. Instead, I banged it against every tantalizing situation. No, I never really broke my abstinence—just as my daughter never really broke the goblet but had many close calls.

And you know, I could tell that my Higher Power was standing near me, guarding the abstinence so graciously given to me. God reached out to catch me whenever I risked falling, just as I had kept a careful eye on my daughter.

My abstinence is so very delicate. I know now that even though I have passed the once-elusive thirty-day mark, I must treat my abstinence with tender loving care and gentleness lest it be broken.

— *South Jacksonville, Illinois USA*

Clear Intention

My husband and I are both abstinent compulsive eaters. To celebrate our tenth wedding anniversary and my fiftieth birthday, we saved for five years to take our dream vacation of a cross-country motorcycle trip.

With the clear intention of staying abstinent, we packed the bike with little clothing; our scale, cups and measuring spoons; and enough abstinent canned food for each of us to have two complete abstinent meals.

Our abstinence took precedence over experiencing the Grand Canyon, the Redwood Forest, Mt. Rushmore, Monument Valley, and everything else that we had waited a lifetime to see.

> *Restocking our canned food at the next town, we never forgot that without abstinence and our Higher Power, this trip would not have been possible.*

Having our food with us allowed us the freedom to stop wherever we wanted at an appropriate time. We picnicked at some of the country's most spectacular spots, enjoying the serenity of being alone.

Restocking our canned food at the next town, we never forgot that without abstinence and our Higher Power, this trip would not have been possible.

Thanking our Higher Power, we made it home after 8,500 miles and five weeks on the road, abstinent and grateful.

— *Oaklyn, New Jersey USA*

CHAPTER FIVE

Abstinence and the Tools

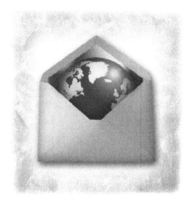

A Choice I Make

Abstinence used to be a tool; now it is a product of working the program. My first abstinence involved eating more food than I do today, but it was a beginning: one breakfast instead of three and no sugary desserts. I soon dropped my mandatory bedtime snack. Eventually it evolved into the simple, one-serving routine I practice today.

I cannot explain how I lost 50 pounds (23 kg) doing that because God did it for me. I cannot lose weight or diet; all I can do is ask God what I should eat today. Then, if I remain willing, I follow through with his plan. I have gained and lost a few pounds since I have been in maintenance. My lowest weight has been 147 pounds (67 kg), and my highest in the last five years has been 157 pounds (71 kg). My usual weight now is 153 pounds (70 kg).

Every day I make a phone call and commit myself to an abstinent day. I do these things as a reminder that I am a compulsive eater and powerless over food, can make and keep commitments one day at a time, and am trustworthy.

No one forces me to commit myself to an abstinent day; it is a choice I make each morning. But electing to choose gives me a good foundation for willingness. If faced with a crazy food thought, I can postpone it until tomorrow: "Well, that's not in the plan today, but if God puts it on the plan tomorrow I can do it then." Guess what?

Diets scare me because instead of being one day at a time, they have multiple-day components—a beginning day and a run for four, seven, fourteen, or twenty-one or more days. Diets imply that when they are over, I can return to "normal" eating, but I can't do that. Put me on a diet, and I immediately start planning to rebel against it, so I make my daily phone call instead.

Some days are more fruitful than others in terms of spiritual or emotional growth. I take at least a few minutes of quiet time a day to think about my day ahead and try to see what it might look like if I "acted as if" I were kind, thoughtful, and unselfish. To help me, I read *For Today, Voices of Recovery*, various daily meditation books, *Lifeline*, OA and AA's "Twelve and Twelve," or the Big Book.

I frequently listen to Twelve-Step tapes or CDs in my car. I meditate and write about the Steps. I study them and see if I can apply them to life's problems in constructive ways.

I try to give service to the meetings I attend. I have routinely attended one to three meetings per week for six years. When I start to rationalize not going to meetings, I get scared. I know from my relapse that I must keep coming back. OA broadly defines service. My service has included showing up, sharing, leading meetings, opening the door, displaying or ordering literature, sponsoring, making and receiving phone calls, attending retreats and intergroup events, being a *Lifeline* rep and a speaker, writing an article for *Lifeline,* giving someone a ride, and acting as treasurer and secretary.

I journal every day, which I swore I would never do. This has provided insight to my character defects and sanity and has helped me accept life on life's terms on most days.

I use the tools of the program and am grateful to be here today, six years abstinent, participating in Step Twelve by carrying the message to all of you that there is a solution.

— *Haymarket, Virginia USA*

Abstinent Sponsors

Abstinence is a commitment, a decision, and an action—of this I am aware. It is a commitment and a decision I made over 34 years ago. I've been taking the actions necessary a day at a time ever since. It has also been a surrender process. The more I surrendered, the more I realized freedom from food obsession. I learned early I would not be able to keep this priceless gift if I didn't share it.

My life began to take on a new meaning. The more I was abstinent, the more I wanted to be abstinent. Abstinent spon-

> *Abstinent sponsors came into my life, sharing with me the need to work the Twelve Steps.*

sors came into my life, sharing with me the need to work the Twelve Steps. I began to learn that this is a spiritual program. Conscious contact with a power greater than me, one that guides me into actions that strengthen my commitment to abstinence, keeps me abstinent over the long haul. By reaching out to an abstinent sponsor, I am putting into action my commitment to abstinence and developing my spirituality. As a result, I live an abstinent life.

I learned that I had to give it back. Sponsorship, Twelfth-Step work, and my relationship with the God of my understanding keep me abstinent. It is important in my abstinent life to practice the OA Twelve Traditions, especially Tradition Five. As our OA Preamble reads, "Our primary purpose is to abstain from compulsive overeating and to carry this message of recovery to those who still suffer." Not only does abstinence allow me to receive a glorious life, it grants me a way to give back. One of the greatest joys of recovery comes to me when I share our OA program with other compulsive overeaters.

The spiritual awareness principle continues to increase my understanding of the necessity of abstinent sponsors. I can't give what I don't have. The knowledge of God's will and the power to carry it out in my life is what gives me the strength to continue my commitment to abstinence and the actions I need to take to carry this life-giving, life-saving message to the next compulsive eater. As *The Twelve Steps and Twelve Traditions of Overeaters Anonymous* taught me, "Those of us who live this program don't simply carry the message; we *are* the message" (p. 106).

I am a grateful, abstinent sponsor. I am aware how important this is. For this I thank God, the OA program, and my beloved Fellowship of Overeaters Anonymous.

— *Houma, Louisiana USA*

Fit Food Around Life

Just like my abstinence and recovery, my action plan has evolved over the years. It began with a dedicated, daily quiet time in the morning. I would read from program daily readers and then talk to my Higher Power about what I needed for my recovery that day. It grew to include many elements, such as a daily reaffirmation of my plan of eating and abstinence; a review of my Tenth Step; a request to remove key character defects; and a request for my HP to show me my day's priorities, coupled with asking for the positive qualities that would help me carry out those actions with sanity and abstinence.

An important part of my action plan is a reminder that I need to fit my food around my life instead of limiting my life because of the food. In my disease I avoided many positive activities because I would rather eat. I needed to be in a "safe" environment so I could "overcontrol" my undereating and weight because my body-image issues made me feel inadequate or I was afraid I would fail if I tried to live a real life. A big part of my recovery involves finding a way to lead a full life without compromising my abstinence.

Every morning I take time to think about today's activities and how I can fit appropriate meals around them. If I have a busy day, it's important to plan healthy, abstinent meals that are easy to prepare so I don't become over-hungry and irritable.

My action plan also includes a balance of other tools. Most important, it includes a sincere attempt to live in the principles of the Steps. This allows me to feel good enough about my behavior and myself so I no longer have to turn to the food for comfort or use it as a means to avoid my life's issues.

I woke up today still feeling off after a challenging day. I asked my Higher Power to help me use my program to be my higher self. Higher Power led me to read my *Lifeline*, the only literature I had handy. I saw the request for an article on action plan, so I started writing before eating an abstinent breakfast. This plan for the day lifted me out of my character defects and allowed me to live my day well.

— *Anonymous*

Hidden Part

I want to eat. I reach for the food, but what am I really reaching for? I am not hungry—not for food. I'm hungry for comfort, warmth, and inner calm. I'm hungry to be loved and have fun. I search for what to do, how to handle my issues and situation—and I reach for the food.

The tools can rescue my sanity and recovery in a moment of need.

But I stop myself. I write this instead. Writing—what a helpful tool! I keep my hands busy and my mind focused on the task before me. I forget the food while my Higher Power provides answers through my writing. Is that the hidden part of the tools I'd never seen? They can rescue me right now.

I knew the tools were central to the program and my recovery in a "big picture" kind of way, but now I see how they can also rescue my sanity and recovery in a moment of need. I call someone, and I don't eat while dialing or talking. I focus on the conversation and get out of my head. I write my thoughts and release the feelings, focusing on my writing and occupying my hands. I do service in any form, which reminds me about the program.

Sometimes when I'm with another OA person and doing a good deed, I feel good about myself. So, how could I eat!

I go to a meeting—no food allowed! I talk to my sponsor, who tells me what I need to hear, and the food goes away without me even realizing it. I read the literature, occupying my hands and mind, focusing on the words of hope and courage. How could I break my abstinence while reading the Big Book, the OA "Twelve and Twelve," or *Lifeline*?

I follow my written food plan; it frees me from thinking about what I'll eat. Doing so allows me to focus on more productive things, like my recovery and life. I remember what it was like before my abstinence, and I do whatever it takes to keep this beautiful gift my Higher Power has provided. I cherish my abstinence.

So, use the tools, whichever you wish and whichever works best for you at that moment. The tools are key to our recovery over time, but they also help keep us abstinent in the moment. The tools are always available. So reach for the tools instead of the food. They are always ready to come to the rescue.

— *Miami, Florida USA*

The Pen Is Mightier Than the Relapse

This morning I find myself at the point where things usually start to go wrong. Following a two-week abstinence and some progress on the scale, I eat a light and abstinent breakfast, and I'm suddenly filled with rebellion and rage. I want to eat! I want to eat more!—for no reason at all.

I'm not really hungry, yet I'm dying to put something in my mouth. At the same time I'm scared, wanting very much to stay abstinent. And I have a strong desire to write.

I sit quietly, take a few deep breaths, and make some tea. As I slowly sip it, I begin writing. I'm holding on now and starting to relax.

I seem to have weathered the storm. I'm calmer, more at peace, feeling better mentally, physically, and spiritually. I'm actually less hungry.

This is a miracle! Still writing, I get the idea of sending this to *Lifeline*. Now I'm feeling humble and infinitely grateful. Thank you, OA!

In trying to understand what just happened, I'm very aware of a great deal of pain connected with the idea of "falling off" my abstinence. I had felt something pushing me on to that precipice with a great deal of force. I still don't understand why it happened, but I'm relieved and grateful for how it turned out.

Writing was my rescuer. One more time, I realized why this is my favorite tool. It's always available, is most accommodating to me and my moods, and provides an excellent record for later perusal—and for reference if a similar crisis strikes in the future. In times of stress I find it easier to write than to dial a phone number.

I'm feeling a hundred percent better now, and I've overcome my desire to jump off my abstinence.

Next, I need to take some effective and constructive action. Typing up the story and hopping on my bicycle to mail it to *Lifeline* will be therapeutic—another phase of my healing.

Thank you, Higher Power, thank you, OA, and thank you, *Lifeline*.

— Palo Alto, California USA

Serenity in A Suitcase

I've traveled quite a bit during the eight years of my OA recovery. At first I couldn't go anywhere without being into the food. But in the last five years I've been given the gift of abstinence on business trips, in the mountains, at the beach, and while visiting family.

Away from home I chose not to make meetings a part of my program. I'd pack my daily meditation books, my journal, my phone book, some weighed and measured food and my Higher Power. I'd keep in touch with my sponsor and OA friends, read program literature, write in my journal, and abstain.

This past winter my husband and I flew to Florida for our yearly visit to my parents. The weather was beautiful, so we retreated on a mini-vacation by ourselves. When we returned to finish our stay with my parents, the pain of my childhood of compulsive eating reared its ugly head.

I was surrounded by lots of food not on my food plan, tireless attention to what I was and wasn't eating, and constant banter about food. What a reminder of the way I lived before recovery!

During those two days I was unable to pick up the phone. It was as though I was trapped in the past. One night I thought: "Okay, I've had enough of this pain, I'm going to eat—things I haven't eaten in six years and lots of them!" I just didn't care anymore.

But my HP took over. As if being led by the hand, I did what's always worked for me during times of intense stress when the food is calling to me: I read program literature and started writing. This story is a result. I had to share the miracle of abstinence. Even though I couldn't call anyone to ask for help, my HP knew I was willing to hear this message.

My HP is always there for me; I just need to listen. As I wrote, I heard the voices of my OA friends, just as if I'd called them, telling me how excess food won't make the pain go away. And the teddy bear I got at the 1992 World Service Convention in Baltimore was sitting on the bed right behind me sending me more messages of abstinence!

In twelve more hours I'll be on a plane back to my OA family. This trip reminded me that I need to take all the tools of the OA program with me when I travel. It helped me see that one hour in a meeting away from home can add one more day of serenity and abstinence to my life.

— *Rockville, Maryland USA*

Taming the Bear

I recently read an account of a fatal bear attack. It was a sad story, but not one which would usually keep me awake at night. But it did. I was struck by how ill-prepared was the victim, and how irrational and persistent the bear.

I'm in my fifth year of program and actively working the Steps to the best of my ability, faithfully attending meetings and sponsoring as well. Lately though my abstinence hasn't been all I want it to be; thoughts of food and bingeing have become more frequent and compelling.

I couldn't put the bear attack out of my mind. I talked it over with an OA friend and discovered I identified with the victim. I felt like a silent witness as she stood alone—helpless, hopeless, unarmed, and defenseless.

> *Because of the Twelve Steps and the Fellowship of OA, I have a number of tools I can use in my defense.*

I can imagine what horror filled her mind in her last moments because, in some measure, I know.

I am that woman, and the bear is my disease. It, too, is irrational. It has nothing to gain from my death, yet it single-mindedly seeks to consume me.

Unlike that unfortunate woman, however, I am not alone and helpless. Because of the Twelve Steps and the Fellowship of OA, I have a number of tools I can use in my defense.

Strongest of these is my Higher Power, always available and only a prayer away. I have my sponsor and my fellow OAs. I have meetings for support, literature for information and inspiration, writing for release and understanding, the telephone and service to get me out of myself.

I can choose to go alone into the wilderness or I can go prepared.

— *Milton, Washington USA*

Sharing Thanks

Thank God I compulsively purchased all the OA literature seven years ago after I returned to OA following a painful three-year relapse. I've been disheartened about OA lately, constantly comparing it to my "old" meetings and finding the new meetings wanting. I moved from Boston to a little town where food-plan meetings are all the rage and Step meetings are scarce.

Early this morning I was melancholy and missing my old, more spiritual meetings. I picked up my *Lifeline Sampler* and read "Visit to a Small Meeting." It's a beautiful story, full of gratitude and abstinence, about a member who is a one-person meeting. It made me realize I should be grateful for my situation. There are Step meetings without food requirements in this area, attended by people with my kind of spiritual life.

But I still miss my Boston meetings. I sat in the same seats three times a week for four years. It will take me a long time to find three comfortable seats here. I miss that gloriously joyous feeling that comes from sharing and hearing others share their practice of the

Twelve Steps. Yet I am confident that feeling will return.

I'm grateful to everyone who ever shared at an OA meeting. Your quest for abstinence and serenity, your sharing and your dumping, your anger and your joy have taught me to live a life without compulsive overeating. I have just celebrated seven years of abstinence. Together we did what I couldn't do alone.

— *Tewksbury, Massachusetts USA*

Following Directions

If insanity is doing the same thing over and over and expecting different results, then sanity then must be doing the same thing over and over and expecting the same results. In the Second Step, I came to believe that a Higher Power could restore me to sanity.

When I came into OA nineteen years ago, I didn't know my thinking was twisted and irrational. All I knew was that I had a 100-pound (45-kg) weight problem, and I couldn't stop eating. I was desperate enough not to argue the insanity issue, but to follow directions. I was to choose a plan for eating and consider myself abstinent if I followed it. Following this plan meant writing the food I would eat for the next day and calling it in to my sponsor. I would make phone calls before picking up the first bite, attend meetings regularly with no excuses, and read literature daily.

The food plan never functioned as a diet for me. It didn't tell me what I was depriving myself of, but what I would eat. The food plan was not punishment, but simply the way any normal, sane human being would nourish his body. It was not something I could look forward to ending—like a diet.

I chose a food plan that OA offered at the time. Even then, I realized the specific foods on the plan were not the important issue. I chose a plan based on what I saw as my food problems. I saw addiction to sugar and to eating as my two big problems. I always wanted to be putting some food, any food, in my mouth. The plan I chose allowed no sugary foods and restricted eating to three meals a day.

That was the road I took to abstinence nineteen years ago, and

I'm on nearly the same road today. I no longer write down specific foods or call them in to a sponsor, although I still follow the same plan. I do more program work. I call my sponsor daily, and I sponsor four members. I follow the original guidelines for food that I chose when I entered OA. I regularly attend two meetings a week, study the Steps and Big Book, and seek to practice the Step principles in all my affairs.

Because of the grace of my Higher Power, I have not binged or relapsed since coming into program. I have faith that continuing to do what has worked these nineteen years will continue to give me the gift of abstinence one day at a time.

— *San Antonio, Texas USA*

My Maintenance Checklist

I've been coming to OA meetings for twenty-two years and am maintaining more than twenty years of abstinence. My top size was thirteen; now I wear sizes eight and ten. The ravages of compulsive eating took me to eating loaves of bread at a sitting, along with entire cakes, bags of cookies, and huge candy bars. Compulsive overeating had me consuming large amounts of laxatives and sticking my fingers down my throat to purge. I stole food from supermarkets to maintain my habit. After a binge, I ran around a race track to complete exhaustion.

When I went to my first OA meeting, the disease had me whipped—physically, financially, emotionally (relationships were out of the question), and spiritually. I had smothered the God of my understanding.

In December of 1979 I became abstinent, willing to stop stealing food and stop bingeing. The purging had stopped a year or so earlier, through prayer. I called my food sponsor and told her I was holding an oversized candy bar in my hand. She asked me if I could throw it away. I did, and that weekend I found a Step sponsor who gave me questions for each Step. I'd write my answers and then call her and read them. I still do this, and I still work the Steps in all areas of my life.

Writing is one of my key tools; it gets me to a place that a conversation never can. I write down my food. If it's a stressful time for me, I call it in to a fellow OA member. I attend one to three OA meetings each week, depending on my schedule. I read *For Today* and pages 86 to 88 in the AA Big Book every morning. I meditate, preferably for twenty minutes, less if that's all I can do. I stay in touch with other OA members; they're some of my dearest friends.

I get OA phone numbers in places I visit. Making a call or going to a meeting can save my sanity. Two years ago I attended a five-day intensive writing workshop in Taos, New Mexico. I was having a difficult emotional time there and went to two OA meetings that week. A lovely woman picked me up and took me there. I would not have made it through without that contact.

I love what this program has given me. I would not be here today without it.

This checklist helps me:

- Find meetings while on vacation.
- Weigh on the same scale every month.
- Call in the food.
- Write every day and read the Tenth Step when necessary.
- Exercise.
- Attend one to two OA meetings weekly and more when you're in trouble.
- Read AA and OA literature every day.
- Seek outside help when necessary, including therapy and other Twelve-Step recovery meetings.
- Avoid recreational sugars: pies, cakes, candies.
- Practice having a peaceful and contented mind. Meditate.

— *Los Angeles, California USA*

Simple Plan

I'm a grateful, abstinent food addict. I have been abstinent and in OA for eight and a half years, maintaining a 100-pound (45-kg) weight loss by the grace of God, the Twelve Steps and the Twelve Traditions.

Staying abstinent while pregnant is simple. I just follow my food plan like I always do. When I first learned I was pregnant, I talked with my sponsor and increased my protein intake, as midwives recommended. I added a snack or two where needed, with my sponsor's guidance. (I've only had to do this early in my pregnancies.) I follow my adjusted food plan and commit it to my sponsor, one day at a time.

> *It's simple: trust God, keep the fork down, and follow my food plan while living a Twelve-Step way of life like I always do.*

Because of God's grace, I have never had any problems in either of my two pregnancies. I've gained a "normal" amount of weight during pregnancy and lost it afterwards (at least with the first pregnancy—I am only three months into my second). If I keep doing what I've been doing, working the OA Twelve Steps and Traditions, God will keep me abstinent. I make sure to use each of the OA tools to help ensure my abstinence.

The biggest food challenge while pregnant is not eating all of my vegetables. I eat as much as I can, leave what I can't, and don't eat anything else. I never eat outside of my three-meals-a-day food plan, unless it's a planned snack during early pregnancy.

It's simple: trust God, keep the fork down, and follow my food plan while living a Twelve-Step way of life like I always do. God will take care of me. He always has and will, no matter what!

— *Waterloo, Iowa USA*

CHAPTER SIX

Abstinent Living

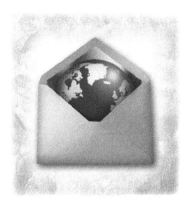

Keeping Food Where It Belongs

When OA found me, I'd never heard of a compulsive overeater. And I didn't know I was one. I did know I was unhappy with my weight and unhappy at work. I would go out each afternoon for a treat to get through the day. I was unhappy at home and would stand many evenings in the kitchen eating ice cream from the container, silently daring my husband to say a word about it. I was furious with God for failing to deliver on my demands, and I would eat out with friends, indulging in complaints and gossip along with appetizers and drinks.

I was intrigued when an acquaintance told me about OA. I wanted to be thin, and I had heard that OA had striking results and, even better, no dues or fees. A local OA meeting was my first introduction to the Twelve Steps, but none of it made sense to me. How could it when I wasn't open to understanding? God couldn't possibly care about my weight; the world had bigger problems.

What did make sense to me was Step Zero. A woman at the meeting demonstrated an "abstinence kit": food scales, measuring cups, a straight-edge ruler, and a telephone. These, she said, were the keys to freedom. I thought she meant freedom from being overweight, so I jumped in with both feet. I got a sponsor, a food plan, a scale, a Big Book, and an OA "Twelve and Twelve." Every day I called my sponsor and committed my food, read the literature, wrote my assignment, and talked to three other OA members. Every week I went to a meeting and did service. Then, and only then, did I begin to understand.

Yes, the weight came off, but by the time I stepped on the scale after my first month, I realized something was going on I could never have imagined. I was beginning to understand that food had never been my problem. It had only been the impenetrable wall I had built between God and me. It had been my reaction to anything in life that made no sense to me. Instead of dealing with my confusion and pain, instead of being honest with myself and asking for help, instead of going to God with my brokenness and being vulnerable, I ate.

I never would have guessed what my problem really was or been open to the answer until I put down the food.

The food has been down for six and a half years. The weight has stayed off for six years. That was why I came to OA, but it's not why I stay. I stay because I have experienced the huge emotional displacements and rearrangements that come with surrender. And every day, I demonstrate my surrender first by keeping the food where it belongs.

— *Twin Cities, Minnesota USA*

I'm Okay

When *Dignity of Choice* first became available, I ran to the back of the meeting room before the closing prayer to buy a copy. I was afraid they would sell out. Even though I had been in program for almost two years and maintained my weight at a size six or eight for several months (I started the program at size ten or twelve), I still wanted to find the magic food plan that would make it easy.

Well, no such thing exists. But the pamphlet did give me validation for the way I already ate. For example, I like to drink warm milk before bed. My family never did this when I was small, no one told me to do it, and I don't remember how I got started. I just know it works for me. Some of the food plans in *Dignity of Choice* have a bedtime meal including one cup of milk or its substitute. When I read this, I felt reassured that what I do is okay.

This is the essence of OA for me: learning I am "okay" and can trust myself (with the guidance of God and a sponsor). The OA "Twelve and Twelve" says, " . . . a source of wisdom inside us . . . becomes more powerful as we recover from compulsive eating and develop our relationship with our Higher Power . . . As we work the steps . . . intuition begins to function properly, helping us focus on God's will, both for our eating and for the living of our lives" (*The Twelve Steps and Twelve Traditions of Overeaters Anonymous*, p. 22).

This confirmed what my intuition had told me, and for that I am grateful.

— *Naples, Florida USA*

What Is "Normal"?

In 1981 I joined OA after reading an article about OA in a newspaper column. I was forty-eight years old and dangerously obese, and I had exhausted every diet between my eleventh and forty-eighth birthdays. I was unhappy, dealing with teenage children, a rocky marriage and most of all, aches and pains caused by my weight.

The one thing that stayed with me was that I would no longer diet; I would get abstinent. And what was abstinence? I am a compulsive overeater. I would eat day in and day out in addition to my three meals a day. No limit existed to my hoarding of food. I would justify it by saying it was on sale.

I was also compulsive about other things, like work. I was an overachiever at school and work. And yet I could do nothing to help myself with my addiction and compulsion.

Someone said, "Why don't you put a picture of yourself at a normal weight on the refrigerator?" Looking back, I had this problem even before I was eleven years old. What is a "normal" weight when one weighs 115 pounds (52 kg) at age eleven? I had to overcome the obsession and compulsion.

I am powerless, so where would this power come from? It had to come from the God of my understanding. The way I prayed had to be different too. I realized God was not going to do for me what I could do for myself. So my biggest prayer became: "God, give me the willingness to abstain, be teachable and work the Steps. God, give me the willingness to forgive and to ask for forgiveness. Give me the willingness to accept myself as I am—as I hope to be." I prayed that God's will would be done in my life.

I used to attend two OA meetings a week. Now I still study and work the Steps; and I talk, walk and sleep the program. I have done all kinds of service. Today I serve by continuing to sponsor, work online with others and do what I can to keep my serenity, abstinence and peace. I am 100 pounds (45 kg) lighter.

What is "normal" weight? Well, it's whatever I'm at today. My marriage is strong, my teenagers have become beautiful adults, and most of all, I am blessed with a purpose in life. I had to go through so much to recognize that God does not make junk! I am precious. For today, I am at normal weight. Thank you, OA. Thank you, God.

— *Ontario, Canada*

So Grateful

I am so grateful for abstinence, no matter what, in my life. I am grateful for my Higher Power, no matter what, in my life. I am grateful for OA, no matter what, in my life.

I just moved 7,000 miles to another continent, from summer to winter, from big city to tiny town. Loads of things have changed, but I'm grateful certain things stay the same: abstinence, Higher Power, and OA. I've been to three meetings in two weeks, found a temporary sponsor here, and reached out often by email to OA members. I slipped into lots of self-centeredness and thoughtless talking, such as saying things without thinking first and hurting people as a consequence.

> *I'm so grateful I continue to grow and improve in this program, even after almost three decades of abstinence.*

I also slipped into controlling behavior, such as wanting people to do things my way and telling folks what they *need* to do. I am so grateful to have a program that reminds me to clean up my act as I go along. Through Step Ten, I've made the amends I need to make. With the help of my Higher Power, I am trying to stay alert to these defects as they arise, or to at least be willing to admit them afterwards and clean up. I am grateful to have a program that reminds me I'm not alone and I don't have to handle this by myself.

Through Step Eleven, I am reaching out to God through prayer and writing, and by sharing with others aloud and on email my need to surrender my perfectionism and to work on things I can improve.

I am grateful to have a program that thrusts me into community.

Through Step Twelve, I have already collected several phone numbers for people at local meetings I've attended, and I've reached out to others whose emails I have with me. These contacts remind me to just keep on keeping on, practicing positive principles, such as acting more thoughtfully and being less self-centered. I'm so grateful I continue to grow and improve in this program, even after almost three decades of abstinence.

— *Anonymous*

If You Work It

To this day, I have been blessed with continuous abstinence. I joined the OA program in September 2004, and my commitment to abstinence began in October of that year. It took me a good four weeks of crash-and-burn incidences with food to recognize I am not normal around food, nor shall I ever be. What a liberation this admission is in my life.

I have just returned home from a short holiday spent in a quiet beach house. Telephone reception was limited; and being blessed with daily phone calls from sponsees and a daily call to my sponsor, I was nervous about this break in routine. I'm thankful a wise member in program reminded me I must pick up the OA tools that are available in any given circumstance, and not just pick them up, but *use* them.

Now back home and having enjoyed several abstinent days away, I realize that this inspired program truly *does* work *if* we work it. The details of how we work it can vary from time to time, but the point is to *work it, no matter what.*

I am also experiencing another level of gratitude for program today. Earlier today, my brother came over and was quite upset. He is facing some unsettling circumstances. Thanks to abstinence, working this program, and finding my Higher Power, I found that God enabled me to be present for my brother—to listen to him and focus my attention without lapsing into self-absorption or ego-driven thoughts of self. And by the grace of God, I was able to share with my brother how the principles embodied in our extraordinary program help me face and deal with life: the people, places, and things that can present daily challenges.

If I was not abstinent today, I could not have been present for my brother because I would have been suffering the anaesthetizing effect of my bingeing food fog or plotting how I was going to cleanse myself of the binge. Either way, when I am in the disease, little room exists for anything or anyone else. Program reinforces that living in active addiction is a full-time job. And thanks to abstinence, OA, God, and members committed to trudging this "Road of Happy Destiny" (*Alcoholics Anonymous*, 4th ed., p. 164) with me, today is another day I am privileged to carry this message of recovery in all of my affairs. The miracle of this simple yet profound program can be a reality for each of us, one day at a time. It *does* work if we work it.

— *Anonymous*

Gains and Losses

Anxious, I have awaited my thirtieth day of abstinence so I would know how great I've been doing! Right? Wrong! I was devastated this morning. I got on that horrible contraption in our bathroom and weighed myself only to find, to my horror, I had only lost 8 pounds (4 kg). How could that be? What did I do wrong? Maybe my scales were broken? No! How could I tell my sponsor? How could I tell my OA group?

> *What more could God give me in only thirty short days?*

I wanted to lose at least 12 to 15 pounds (5 to 7 kg) per month. At this rate it will take me a year to reach my goal weight! But why do I feel so thin? Why do I feel so light and good? As the hurt, anger and frustration left my mind, heart and soul, a feeling of peace and serenity entered, and I came to these realizations:

I have lost that heavy, dense, black cloud in my mind. I have lost the horrible, heavy burdens from my shoulders. (I have carried them day after day, needlessly, unable to do anything with them.)

I have lost the heavy feeling in my heart. I have lost the feelings of sadness, gloom, self-hate, doubt and darkness. I have lost over 7 inches (18 cm). My bra no longer leaves big, red marks. My "big" clothes fit again. My body is willing to move.

I've lost only 8 pounds (4 kg)? Well, I have gained a way of living that brings me closer to my Higher Power. I now have a life that gives me peace, joy, happiness, serenity, and friends. What more could God give me in only thirty short days? I thank my Higher Power, my sponsor, and my OA group. I am grateful.

— *Mesa, Arizona USA*

This Girl's Tale

Seventeen years ago, this girl walked into her first OA meeting. She had reached 248 pounds (112 kg) some time back, and the solution was to stop weighing herself. Unfortunately, that didn't stop her uncontrolled binges, and she went up another dress size. She had considered taking her own life, but then a friend took her to an OA meeting.

She scanned the tables for the "diet" but found none. The concepts were foreign—get a sponsor, take the Steps and call three people a day. None of the sponsors was available, so what could she do? But for the first time in a long time, she had hope. OA was not like diet clubs. Most of the OA women had normal body sizes. Some were fat like her, but even what they shared sounded hopeful!

At the end of the meeting, they gave out poker chips for abstinent people. What did "abstinent" mean? She knew she must have one of those white chips because she was tired of her life. She wanted to be a member of this club.

The following night she went to another OA meeting. This time a woman said she was a sponsor and did not say she was unavailable. After the meeting she asked the woman to be her sponsor. The woman agreed and told her to call the next day and not eat any sugar. Bizarre as it was, she did it; and life, as she knew it, was over.

With her sponsor, she jumped into the Steps. She thought she'd try the Twelve-Step, twelve-week plan, graduate, and never be fat again. So each week she talked to her sponsor about a Step. By the fifth week, she was on Step Five, losing weight at a good clip, and answering all the questions from *The Twelve Steps of Overeaters Anonymous* (the Traditions part had not yet been written).

Over time she learned it doesn't work that way. We don't graduate. It is a lifelong process, one day at a time. "Whatever," she thought, but did everything her sponsor suggested. As time went on, 100-plus pounds (45-kg) of excess weight melted away. She understood more about how OA worked because her life felt so much better than before. She'd arrive early at meetings, help put out chairs and talk to newcomers.

A girl at the meeting got a ninety-day abstinence chip. Wow! If that girl could do it, so could she! Today, she still goes to OA meetings and has a normal body size. She has had several different sponsors over the years. She has taken the Steps several times over, and her food plan has changed many times. Now when they ask for sponsors, she always raises her hand. She has been chairwoman of an OA region and knows that doesn't make her important. She is just another bozo on the bus, and giving back is important.

She loves her life again, and people love her. Unlike those diet clubs, OA helped her understand why she ate like that. When she reached a normal body size, she didn't have to celebrate at a doughnut shop. No, she quietly wrote this story, hoping it would help another compulsive overeater who still suffers. She puts her abstinence first, absolutely. Today she cares about others.

I celebrate my abstinence through God's grace and your help! I am grateful to all who've walked this path with me. I'm no longer a woman who abuses food. I like who I am today—can you believe it? I think I'll keep coming back.

— *Titusville, Florida USA*

Finding the Miracle

I am one of many who joined OA just to lose weight. I wasn't a compulsive overeater. I just liked food—plenty of sweet, gooey food.

I was a sickly, emaciated child until I was six. After that I was usually five to 10 pounds (2 to 5 kg) overweight. But it didn't bother me because I was a successful dieter. Of course, I'd gain it back plus more once the diet ended.

When my mother (my guru) died, I had to gather her things from two states outside my home state. Added to this were my on-call 24/7 career of mother and wife and grief over my loss. I was about to get sick when I remembered my mother's advice during my teenage fasting diet: "You have to eat to keep up your strength." I kept up my strength over 200 pounds (100 kg). How much over I don't know, since I wouldn't weigh myself.

After twenty-eight years in OA, even I am amazed at the difference in me.

My diet buddy retired in July when we were both at our goal weights. At an office "pig-out," she arrived still slim; I was bursting out of a size 22. My plate was heaping while hers was abstinent. I asked about her diet, and she told me about OA.

I had a friend in AA, so I knew the Twelve Steps worked. She helped me find a home group, and I jumped in compulsively. I bought all the literature, got a sponsor, started working the Twelve Steps, got abstinent and lost 30 pounds (14 kg). My problem with OA was that it took away the time I used to spend with my husband, eating. So I thought I had the knowledge and literature and could do it on my own. Six months and 25 pounds (11 kg) later, I realized I couldn't. In relapse, I returned to the rooms and started to serve compulsively until I found I had been elected Miss OA, doing all the work. I fell off that pedestal and spent three months in relapse. Again I gained 15 pounds (7 kg). My last relapse (and I mean last) occurred because I was alone for three consecutive weeks, poor me. If they couldn't be there for me, I wouldn't be there for them. One month and 10 pounds (5 kg) later, I got the message that this is a "me" program. I have to do this for me. I must never relapse again.

Before OA I was cynical, vengeful, grudge-carrying, suicidal, but always smiling and people pleasing. I made plenty of money calming stormy waters at work, but the rest of the time I was a terror. I never believed in an eye for an eye; it was a head for an eye. I was a master of sarcasm, never having met the person I couldn't bring to his knees with my sizeable vocabulary and razor-sharp tongue. OA taught me that my righteous indignation was merely resentment. That was a shock. I thought my unhappiness was my husband's fault. One day while repeating the Serenity Prayer, I finally heard it. I was the one staying in a situation I hated. Either I left or stayed with a smile.

I never intended to leave, so at last I had my serenity.

After twenty-eight years in OA, even I am amazed at the difference in me. Gone are the 60 pounds (27 kg) of excess weight, never to return. Gone is the cynicism. Life is life. Gone are vengefulness and sarcasm. Things just don't make me mad now. Gone are grudges and resentments. They are in the past, and I played a part too. Gone is the urge to commit suicide while driving; now I'm careful. What remains is the smile, because now I allow myself to be happy. Added is an occasional frown because I allow myself to feel pain; it is no longer stuffed down with food.

One of our favorite sayings is "OA is simple, but it isn't easy." As an independent person, I had to learn to trust, listen to, and lean on a sponsor. The least I can do is go to meetings. Abstinence is number one, and I can't stay abstinent without the help of my Higher Power, sponsor and fellow OAers. Making a plan of eating and action plan and sticking to them with the help of God, my sponsor, and fellow OAers have brought me the miracle. Don't leave until you have it. Then stay for the fun of it.

— *Fayetteville, Tennessee USA*

Right Now

"You can get down on your knees and ask for help right now." That's what someone in OA wrote to me many years ago when I had written that things were hard. I'm glad she did, and I'm glad I did. Oh, I had plenty to complain about: living in a community with no phones, electricity, or running water in a country where I didn't speak the local language. She reminded me that any day can be our first day or next day of abstinence. That's an amazing fact in OA.

I'm grateful for my abstinence and wouldn't want to live without it. Abstinence means I have lots of work to do each day to work the Step I'm on. I completed Step Nine 22 years ago and am working Steps Ten, Eleven, and Twelve today. Each day is a miracle! Each day is a day I want to stay well, so I do whatever I must do to work my Steps: contact a sponsor when needed (which I did daily for many years), write, read literature, work with newcomers and others working the first nine Steps, and write letters to OA folks.

As the Big Book says, this can work for anyone who has "the capacity to be honest" (*Alcoholics Anonymous,* 4th ed., p. 58). For me that means looking at my defects that arise each day; moving through the Tenth Step; and getting out of myself by forcing myself to think of someone to help, usually by being abstinent one more day.

Today you, like me and everyone in OA, have a choice to pick up the food or not. I hope you choose a sane and abstinent day, no matter how hard it feels. Today that's my choice.

— *Australia*

An Abstinent Vacation

Our vacation of a lifetime had been in the works for nearly six months, well before I was introduced to OA. Now, only two months abstinent, I was preparing to leave on a week-long adventure aboard a sixty-five foot sailboat in the Bahamas. We were planning to enjoy a week of scuba diving and sailing—no phones, no TV, no alarm clocks. I was faced with a week of being out in the middle of the ocean with very limited food options.

> *I know that I can deal with my feelings today without shoving something in my mouth.*

Determined to stick to my food program, I called the cruise office to discuss my needs. I was assured that special consideration would be extended, and there would be no problem. I called again a few days later to hear a similar reassurance.

The week before we left, I attended every available OA meeting. While taking every precaution, I was acutely aware of how cunning, baffling, and powerful my disease is. To be stranded in the middle of nowhere with minimal food choices was frightening.

Finally the big day arrived. I was armed with my measuring cups, scales, and scads of literature, including, of course, a few copies of *Lifeline*. But as we drove to the port in Miami, I couldn't dismiss my fear. I used the biggest tool available to me: I prayed. As I talked with my Higher Power and "let it go," I felt calmer and knew that somehow everything would be all right.

Once on board I stopped the first crew member I found and asked to be directed to the galley. I explained that I was the passenger who would be the pain in the neck concerning meals.

"Don't worry about anything," he said with a soft smile. "The cook puts up with me, and I'm a recovering alcoholic." I couldn't believe my ears. He introduced me to the cook who confided she, too, was in recovery in another Twelve-Step program.

What a vacation this turned out to be! I explained my food program to the cook, and she weighed, measured, and served every one of my meals. Total abstinence! We found one more friend of Bill W. and the four of us watched the sun rise every morning, sipping coffee and sharing in a very casual Twelve-Step meeting.

I know that I can deal with my feelings today without shoving something in my mouth. One day at a time at home, work, or even on vacation, I have my Higher Power, the tools, and the Twelve Steps to help me live my life. I celebrated ninety days of abstinence last week.

— *Orlando, Florida USA*

Sweet Surrender

There I was, sober and abstinent for three years, back to normal in body weight, involved with daily meetings in South Bend, working closely with my sponsor, and depending on all the tools for sanity. Then my boss offered me a six-week job checking transmission lines in northwestern Pennsylvania. A new truck, video equipment, and a computer would help me cover fifteen miles of line daily. Sounded almost like a vacation.

A miraculous truce with food followed me every step of the way.

But on the first day I was shocked to discover I would have to hike twelve to fourteen miles over rugged terrain just to cover a measly six miles of line in one day, Monday through Saturday. To inspect 490 miles (789 km) of power lines would take four months, through fall and early winter.

The job was impossible. I couldn't possibly finish it. Would I break a leg in the middle of a forest? Be shot by drunken hunters? Mauled by wild dogs? Drowned in a swamp?

Worst of all none of the towns I stayed in was larger than Mishawaka, Indiana, and few people had even heard of OA.

I missed breakfast the first day because my boss refused to stop before reaching the site. I hiked four miles across rivers, fields, and pastures before sitting down to lunch at a greasy diner in Conneautville.

I was hungry. But, by the grace of God, I didn't binge. I ate an abstinent lunch. I didn't allow the circumstances to become an excuse for bingeing.

For two weeks I lost weight and starved between meals. I ate bigger portions but nothing inappropriate. I didn't crave my binge foods. One night I finished a big dinner in Meadville and felt like vomiting. Choking back tears, I headed for the phone in the lobby. Thank God my sponsor was home. I felt I had binged, even though I hadn't. "I want to cut my food intake," I cried.

"If you cut down you'll set yourself up for a real binge," my sponsor replied. "Your body needs the fuel, but your stomach is too small to stoke the furnace. Go slow, don't skip, pray, and get to a meeting."

I discovered how the Steps and tools can help me no matter where I am. The area had many strong Twelve-Step meetings where I met new friends, even some OA members. Calling my recovery friends back home helped so much, too. I pored over my emergency stack of *Lifelines* whenever I felt vulnerable to insanity and isolation.

I learned how to zoom through forests, navigate around and through swamps, jump electric and barbed wire fences, climb Allegheny mountain trails and crisscross timber, oil, and corn country. I had no partner so I had to hike down-line for a mile or two and backtrack to the truck alone.

Soon I noticed that my meals were all consistent. Body weight and size returned to normal and stayed constant. I felt healthy and energetic. All of this without trying to manage the food. A miraculous truce with food followed me every step of the way.

The real crisis was accepting my job and my life in Pennsylvania. Would I finish? Would the boss crucify me for mistakes? Would I break the $3,000 equipment they made me haul cross-country? When would I fall in love and live happily ever after?

I found a meeting in Meadville and a member talked to me afterwards. "Sounds like you're fighting the program. You're making meetings, calls, inventories, prayers, and all that, but you're not letting go. Are you having fun yet?"

"Fun?" I stared at him like an idiot.

"Yes, fun. If you don't turn it over and surrender all your problems to God, how long do you expect to remain sober?"

My first surrender in a long time occurred soon after. I was hiking through a lowland woods in the pouring rain. Switches whipped my face as I struggled through dense, thorny brush. I had to videotape a tower for the second time, and I was angry. I have three degrees, talent, ambition, and ability. Why was I trudging through the woods counting poles?

Then the Serenity Prayer came to mind, and for once I asked God to help. I said aloud the things I had trouble accepting: cold rain, soaked boots, the woods, a crazy job, and loneliness. Could I accept all these for one morning? An enormous burden fell from my shoulders. I felt at peace with myself. Finishing my task in harmony with the way things were became a joy.

For the rest of that day anxiety, obsession, and depression didn't take hold. Food and alcohol held all the appeal of rat poison to me. Every day left on the job I surrendered. When I finally returned home, my portion sizes returned to normal. With God's help, impossible conditions became possible, one day at a time.

— *South Bend, Indiana USA*

Moving Ahead

After eleven years of abstinence, I'd like to share with the readers of *Lifeline* a few insights I have learned on this journey of recovery.

- The food was just a symptom of a deeper problem and served as a "cover-up" for my inner turmoil. With the food in its proper perspective, I must continually work on myself.
- I have feelings. They come and go and are constantly changing. I don't need to do anything about them—I just need to allow them to be. I don't need to let them control my behavior. Being in a bad mood doesn't mean I can be crabby to others.

- This is a twenty-four-hour-a-day program. I need to be on guard for negative thoughts, fear, selfishness, and self-pity. I need to pray for their removal and forgive myself when I indulge in them.
- Constant work on my self-esteem is the key to long-term recovery. Self-hatred kept me in my disease. If I love myself, love others, and love God, I will be more willing to go to any length for freedom from the food compulsion.
- No matter how many days of abstinence I rack up, I still need to share what's going on in my life with my sponsor and other OA friends. Just listening to others and sitting without speaking at meetings won't keep me well. I must open my heart.
- It's very important that I work on being on good terms with others. Hatred, resentment, and judgment hurt only me. The only way to be free from those emotional terrors is to live one day at a time.
- Self-honesty is essential to getting along with others in this world. Without stepping on others' toes, I need to check within to determine what I want in any given situation and express that. It just doesn't work for me to people-please, because I end up resenting the person or myself.
- Abstinence is the most important thing in my life without exception. It must be safeguarded and cherished. How can I do that? By working all of the Steps every day and sharing my experience, strength, and hope with others.

I have grown and changed more in the last eleven years than in the previous twenty. Thanks to OA, the Steps, and this wonderful Fellowship, I have a chance to have a fulfilling and meaningful life. Thanks to all of you for that gift.

— *Oakland, California USA*

Recovery Roster

I know I'm in recovery because:

- I abstain from my trigger foods and have maintained my abstinence and weight loss for five and a half years.
- I stop eating when my body's had enough.
- I've quit weighing myself all the time.
- I go to social functions for the company of the people who'll be there and not for the huge amounts of food.
- Others can eat my binge foods in front of me, and I don't feel resentful; I can prepare my binge foods for others and not even be tempted to lick my fingers.
- I can live within my financial means, even when meager.
- Though disabled, I accept my health limitations without crabbing about them continually.
- Instead of thinking about what I don't have, I'm truly grateful that I have so much.
- I don't make excuses to get out of going to meetings. Unless my health restricts me, I go whether I want to or not.
- I take the time to write, make phone calls, talk to my sponsor, and read OA literature, no matter how much I'd rather be doing something else.
- I can talk to my teenage son calmly when he's in the middle of a temper tantrum.
- When someone hurts me, I don't hold a grudge. I pray, let go, and let God.
- I recognize my character defects and am aware of how they hurt me and other people.
- I realize I can't always have my own way.
- I set healthy boundaries. I don't let people use me as a doormat, nor do I build walls that isolate me.

- I stay out of other people's business and let them run their own lives.
- Instead of "fixing" people I try simply to listen to them, sharing my experience, strength, and hope.
- I eliminate guilt and shame from my life, instead of merely saying, "That makes me feel guilty," and continuing to drag the guilt feelings around with me. I let the past go.
- I don't beat myself up when I make a choice that's not in my best interest; I learn from experience.
- I've stopped being a victim and started being a survivor.
- I accept being a grown-up and take responsibility for changing my actions and attitudes.
- I don't rely on anyone to make me happy, but realize that happiness comes from accepting God's will in my life.

— *Montague, Michigan USA*

Present for Life

As I write this, I'm spending my vacation in sunny Florida with my family. This would be enviable, except for the reason I'm here. Three days ago, my mother and I received a call that my grandmother had taken very ill and might die at any time. So here I sit, looking at the ocean while one of my closest relatives lies in the other room, dying.

I'm twenty-four years old. I've been abstinent almost two years, and I've seen my share of difficulties and accomplishments. I've been accepted at the university of my dreams, but all I can think about is graduation without granny.

This morning I sat on her bed, and we planned the colors for my wedding and what my dress should look like. Neither of us cared that I'm years away from that ceremony.

I'm grateful today for so many things, and I would like to share that gratitude with others—especially the newcomer who can't imagine being abstinent past today.

I'm incredibly grateful for not having my head in the fridge and my face in the toilet. Abstinence has allowed me to be here for my family and for granny. Before I left for Florida, my sponsor reminded me that a quick summary of the Steps is "to grow up." For the first time, I feel very much a part of this family. They've included me in all the talks about granny's condition and have never treated me like a child.

I'm grateful I was able to say things to granny, and she was able to really hear and feel my love for her. If I were eating and throwing up, I'd be stuffing those feelings with tons of food. Five or ten years from now, I'd wish that I'd been able to tell her what she's meant to me. These feelings are very painful, but at last I can feel them. That means I'm really alive.

During the past couple of days, the compulsion has certainly been there. But my HP gives me the strength to deal with what may happen in the next twenty-four hours. I'm grateful for my concept of a loving HP, who promises me that granny is going some place even more beautiful and peaceful than I could ever wish for her.

Thank you, *Lifeline*, OA, and HP for guiding me along a road of recovery to a place where I can support others as well as take care of my own needs.

— *San Diego, California USA*

Finding the Balance

Before finding OA, I didn't know the meaning of the word "balance," and I didn't know that my life was unmanageable. I viewed the world in black-and-white extremes: Everything was either wonderful or awful, perfect or a total disaster. People were either good or bad, and I loved them or hated them. I was either wealthy or poverty-stricken, and of course, if I wasn't thin, I was fat.

And those misguided people in Overeaters Anonymous! Whenever I'd suggest one of my "perfect" solutions at a meeting, they'd debate and discuss it, and usually reject it. Like the time I suggested we use a non-Conference-approved book. When they turned down my sage advice, I was hurt, upset, and just plain mad!

Yet I kept going to meetings. There was nowhere else for me to go. I'd tried controlling my compulsive eating in many ways: diets, diet pills, rewards for losing weight (also known as compulsive spending), and starving. I'd lose weight, then put it back on plus more. I knew OA had answers for me because the people there said I had a disease. They said that I wasn't a bad person trying to become good, but a sick person trying to become well.

Today I find that discussing differences of opinion helps me grow. At first when people in my OA group said, "Take what you like and leave the rest," I thought, "Yeah—I take it that you're crazy, and I'm leaving!" Now I'm learning to separate issues from personalities. Today it's okay for me to have opinions, values, and boundaries, and for others to have differing ones. It's also okay for me to change my ideas, and, later on, change them again.

Before OA I always thought I'd be happy "when." When I get thin. When I get married. When I get divorced. When I get a good job and make lots of money. When I retire. The "when" list went on and on.

Before OA I lived in grief, depression, disappointment, guilt, shame, and despair over past events. I decided I had to work the Steps because I wanted the pain to go away.

Black-and-white thinking was one way I made my life unmanageable. Seeing the world in extremes kept me from people and from myself. Most of all, it kept me from having an intimate relationship with my Higher Power.

Today I can choose to go through problems rather than avoid them, seeing them as opportunities for growth. I recognize this world and the people in it as conduits through which my Higher Power contacts me.

Through OA I've found a way to be happy now. Call it whatever you want; acceptance, balance, growing up, "living life on life's terms." I call it being abstinent, in contact with my Higher Power, and living one day at a time.

— *Crystal Lake, Illinois USA*

Feeling Full

As an abstinent compulsive overeater, I always enjoy being comfortably hungry before each meal, and the feeling of satisfaction afterward. Occasionally I don't feel particularly hungry at mealtimes, but I eat anyway, because that's the best way I can maintain my three-meals-a-day abstinence.

But then there are rare times when I'm so full of feelings, generally negative ones, that I simply don't want to eat. Food tastes like cardboard and feels like a lead ball in my stomach—as if whatever I've eaten is too much and won't ever be digested.

I'm experiencing one of those times right now. I'm so focused on what might happen this coming weekend that I'm having trouble enjoying the richness of each moment and the miracle of abstinence at work in my body and my life.

Food tastes like cardboard and feels like a lead ball in my stomach—as if whatever I've eaten is too much and won't ever be digested.

I think the sensation of being "full of feelings" is a phenomenon unique to abstinence. I've been 60 pounds (27 kg) overweight and 50 pounds (23 kg) underweight at different times in my adult life. When I was anorexic, I was literally starving all the time. It wasn't that I ever had a moment when I didn't want to eat; I simply couldn't eat because I was so terrified of the food and the bingeing I knew I was capable of. Sure enough, self-starvation always led to uncontrollable bingeing, stuffing myself way beyond capacity and yet never feeling full. Or if I felt full, it certainly didn't affect my desire to eat more.

I'm grateful for the support of a wonderful sponsor and friends in the OA program who are there to listen to me and keep me grounded as I experience different levels of recovery. I'm grateful for my own willingness to listen to all my different hungers and the ability to differentiate between my body's needs and my disease, which tells me I'm too "full of feelings" to have room for healthy and abstinent meals.

I've spent the afternoon unraveling some of those feelings, working a few of the appropriate Steps, and topping off my work with this article. As a result, I feel better about myself and have no intention of depriving myself of a delicious, well-balanced supper—or, better yet, a well-balanced life!

— *Washington, D.C. USA*

Party Plan

I was having a battle with myself, trying to decide whether or not to go to a kitchenware party. Parties like that tend to focus on the desserts served afterward.

The guests gather around the overflowing table. A lot of attention is paid to who baked what and who's consuming it. And there's always a fuss made over those who choose not to eat. That lonely and isolated feeling is one I didn't want to experience.

After calling the hostess—a friend who is in another Twelve-Step program—I decided to go to the party. She told me that there wouldn't be great quantities of food on display, and I could leave to consume my planned abstinent meal.

At the party I let myself laugh and enjoy a game, not concentrating on the food items we shouted out as we played. It felt great to be with people I cared about, and I could feel their love for me as well.

But my happiness changed to anger as I revealed some of my current eating habits to a woman sitting next to me, a member of another Twelve-Step program. She was astonished to find that I choose not to eat certain foods and that I weigh and measure what I eat. (I knew most of the volume capacities of the containers being sold!) Her repeated exclamations of "You're so good. You never bake? You're so good!" stimulated my anger.

I told her that it has nothing to do with being "good"—it's what's necessary for me to stay abstinent. I knew she didn't understand. As I was putting on my coat, she asked, "Doesn't it bother you to look at that dessert over there?" I replied, "Of course it bothers me, but it's my choice not to eat it and that's the best choice I can make."

I made a call when I got home. As I expressed my anger to a fellow compulsive eater, I began to cry. There's no way to get around the sense of loss I feel now that I'm abstinent. The sadness from missing the food and the emptiness from feeling different are there. But as long as I feel those feelings and don't pick up the food, I'll make it through another day.

I've worked hard to be blessed with a program that fills me with love. And if going through the pain is what it takes to stay in recovery and to help others, then so be it.

While taking my inventory that night, I recalled this woman had made oblique references to her own problems with overeating. It may be that exclaiming over my lifestyle was a way of denying her own experiences with food. Who knows? I fell asleep wondering if perhaps, without realizing it, I'd planted a seed.

— *Naugatuck, Connecticut USA*

The Tempest

A week ago our island of Kauai was devastated by a hurricane. I have to use the tool of writing today, since I am temporarily without regular meetings, my sponsor, and OA friends.

I waited twenty minutes at our OA meeting room (now converted to a Red Cross headquarters!), praying for someone to show up. As I drove away, I circled the block one last time and saw two OA friends walking towards the meeting room. We found a quiet place and had an OA meeting.

I was comforted to hear that they, too, were being urged to eat trigger foods and oversized, fatty meals by well-meaning friends and neighbors; they, too, had been tempted by offers of ice-cold beer and soda (we have to boil drinking water and very few people have any refrigeration); they, too, were committed to abstinence in a time of high stress and little choice of food and drink; they, too, struggled with honesty while filling out claim forms.

All the old justifications for compulsive overeating—eat now, there might not be food tomorrow; eat more, you need your strength; eat the rest, you can't afford to waste anything—were running amok in their minds, too. They, however, had made it to a meeting despite losing their homes and vehicles in the hurricane.

Life has changed drastically this week. But God still guides me. I have abstinence. I have the Fellowship of OA. I have everything I need to make it through the day.

— *Kauai, Hawaii USA*

The Ghost of Christmas Past

The holidays have always been a dismal time of year for me, mainly because my father died eight days before Christmas when I was nineteen. For most of my life, my father and I weren't very close due to his alcoholism. During the last year of his life, however, he was recovering in AA both emotionally and spiritually, and I came to know him as the caring and loving person he could be.

When he died, I felt that my Higher Power had taken away the father I had always wanted. Through the Twelve Steps of OA, I have come to realize that my HP had given me a wonderful gift—a short period of good times that left memories I can treasure the rest of my life.

Another aspect of Christmas past I've had to deal with is my attitude toward food. Before OA the only thing I looked forward to at Christmas was unrestricted eating. It was the one time of the year I could eat the way I wanted to and not feel guilty. In fact, I felt that gorging myself on seasonal goodies was the expected behavior. I know better now, but it doesn't make abstinence easier.

During my first abstinent Christmas, I struggled to keep away

> *During my first abstinent Christmas, I struggled to keep away from the binge foods of the season.*

from the binge foods of the season. I knew from my Fourth Step that I would be in for a rough time but followed my sponsor's advice to "go to meetings, pray, and not pick up that first compulsive bite." I stayed away from all social functions except for OA and AA, and even then I was cautious. I fought my toughest battles at work where there seemed to be an abundance of seasonal binge foods. To add to the torment, it appeared that everyone at work was attempting to force the junk on me against my wishes. I made it through that period abstinently, one day at a time, with the help of OA and my HP. I now realize that it was nothing more than white-knuckle abstinence.

My second holiday season in OA was a much easier and more enjoyable experience. I used the same Steps and tools that had kept me abstinent the rest of the year. The old binge foods were plentiful as ever but not an issue anymore. I sincerely didn't want any and felt good about it.

I was doubly grateful for the program when I noticed a colleague attempting to diet during the holiday season. Her struggle with food was the same as mine had been the previous year. What struck me most, however, was the look in her eyes. Although she was saying "No, thank you," with her mouth, her eyes were saying, "Please, give me some." I then fully comprehended the state of mind I had been in the previous Christmas. I now have an even greater appreciation for the gift I've been given by God and OA.

Coming up on my third Christmas in program, I'm full of excitement and hope. I'm taking a couple of beginner courses at the local community college, my work is more challenging and rewarding than I expected, I served as a delegate to Region 7 for my intergroup, and so far I've maintained my weight loss and my abstinence. None of this would be possible without HP and OA. I give credit to my sponsors who keep me honest and on an even keel.

I can't guarantee that I won't relapse tomorrow, next week, or next month, but I know what works for me and I'm grateful. This doesn't mean that my life always runs smoothly or that I'm a model of serenity, but it does mean that when I have to confront problems in my life, food is no longer an option.

— *Annapolis, Maryland USA*

An OA Lexicon

How do I know when I've broken my abstinence? How do I tell the difference between relapse, slips, and simple weight gain?

My general rule for identifying slips is eating when I'm not hungry or eating inappropriate food when I am hungry.

I also distinguish between overeating, compulsive eating, and compulsive overeating.

Overeating is when I feel fine but the food tastes so good I eat more than I need. Or when I find it hard to say no to food that is offered to me. I realize that noncompulsive overeaters sometimes overeat too. Simple overeating can make me as fat as compulsive overeating, so it's important for me to think of ways I can protect myself against such situations or to counter overeating at one meal by eating less at my next one.

Compulsive eating is when I swallow my feelings with food. I don't eat more than I should, and I don't eat anything that I consider unhealthy; but I don't process my feelings, I devour my food. I often think about one food while eating another.

Compulsive overeating is a problem of both what and why I'm eating. Mentally and emotionally I'm not okay, and so I try to solve my problems with food.

After many years of abstaining from compulsive overeating, I recently slipped. I was at a social event where I knew only the host and hostess, and feelings of alienation and inadequacy surfaced. Instead of reaching out to the other guests, I embraced the hors d'oeuvres. Not only was I overwhelmed with feelings, but my suffering was compounded by the feeling of heaviness the morning after. Although I had dulled my clarity, a corner of my sane self stayed with me, and I was ashamed at having been out of control.

Writing about the experience made me realize the benefits of the abstinence I had taken for granted. But the price of this realization was too high. I don't want to revisit my pain in order to remember how awful it was. I would rather my slip hadn't happened, but it did happen; and I dealt with it by telling my group about it when I took my fourteen-year candle.

If I'm in relapse, I don't talk about it. I compound the problem by beating myself up. I refuse to take remedial action. I refuse to learn from it, and I continue to sabotage myself by not reaching out. I've given up. I cooperate with my craziness. Relapse starts long before I take that first compulsive bite. It begins with the stinking thinking of cockiness or low self-esteem. It ends with increasing isolation and weight gain.

Simple weight gain is due to physical causes such as medication or eating something with more calories than I can assimilate. Sometimes it happens when my food intake remains the same but I curtail my exercise because of sickness or scheduling. Whatever the cause, I deal with it.

— *Hawthorne, California USA*

Island Oasis

I went to my first OA meeting three and a half years ago with two dreams. The first was to stop compulsively overeating, the second was to travel. So far in recovery, I've kept off 13 pounds (6 kg) and been around the world.

After eighteen months in the program, I had lost 10 pounds (5 kg) and had just landed a new job teaching college-level English to members of the navy—while deployed on a tender taking care of combat ships in the Persian Gulf! As I prepared to leave the States, I had no idea what to expect nor even what coun-

> *She smiled and tapped her daily meditation book. "My Higher Power is really helping me out," she said.*

tries my ship would be visiting as that information was classified. The only instructions I got were that I couldn't wear skirts on board!

Naturally, I was sad to leave my wonderful home OA group, my sponsors, and the members I was sponsoring, but I planned to take my program with me. I'd heard that many ships had Twelve-Step meetings (usually AA) nightly, but I suspected that my classes would probably meet in the evenings, too, when the sailors were off duty. I worried about whether I'd be able to make the meetings, and whether I could work an OA program with only AAs for support. In typical fashion, I found myself worrying needlessly about the following month's schedule of a ship on the other side of the world!

The flight to the Philippines took nineteen hours. After a brief rest, I got onto a military plane full of sailors, and we headed for our next stop, Diego Garcia. Diego Garcia is a tiny island seven degrees south of the equator in the middle of the Indian Ocean. As we landed, the island looked like a scene from *South Pacific:* a coconut grove bordering a clean white beach curving around a horseshoe-shaped bay. We were dying to get in the water, but everyone from the plane had to wait in a huge processing room. There were sailors from dozens of ships, and everyone's paperwork had to be processed in the maddeningly slow way of the military.

In the midst of hundreds of blue and white uniforms, I happened to take a seat behind a woman just as she opened her briefcase to reveal OA pamphlets! I leaned forward and whispered, "I think we have something in common—I'm a compulsive overeater." She smiled and tapped her daily meditation book. "My Higher Power is really helping me out," she said. "I was praying to meet someone here." Amazingly, it turned out that we were en route to the same ship.

We planned to attend an AA meeting together that night on Diego Garcia. I needed one. The temperature was over 100 degrees and the bay that had looked so inviting turned out to be only two feet deep and as warm as the air. After a day of walking in the jungle, fighting off the fat, ferocious mosquitoes and paddling in two feet of hot water, I refused a few invitations to the officers' club and took my sunburned body to the AA meeting.

There were three other people there as delighted to see us as we were to see them, as they don't get many visitors. The island is notoriously boring for people stationed there and heavy drinking is the main activity. The three men we met that night were struggling to recover in the midst of that insanity—and doing a good job.

Once I reached my ship I learned that the AA meetings were held at 8 p.m., right in the middle of my classes. But my shipmate and I started an OA group that met whenever we felt the need—often every day!

Navy ships, I soon discovered, are noisy and crowded places with a lot of unhappy people packed much too close together. This crew had been out to sea for four months, not even catching a glimpse of land for more than sixty days. Low morale showed everywhere. Meals in the officers' wardroom were depressing and silent (I was never tempted to prolong them), and my students, though eager to learn, were exhausted by the endless work of supporting the smaller ships.

Worst of all, we were at anchor, and the ship's weak air conditioning was no competition for the sun baking our metal ship. Some of my students worked in the engine room in 140-degree heat. The temperature on deck, where a few of us sweated through aerobics, was usually 110 to 120 degrees. Down below in the crew's berthing, the heat was barely tolerable. After teaching, I would go on deck in search of a little coolness, but the night air was as hot as the day's.

Because no alcohol was allowed on board, sugar was the drug of choice. In every office or shop I'd see sailors munching sweet junk food. The supply chief told me that one of his biggest problems was keeping the ship stocked with sodas since the 1,100-person crew each drank an average of five cans a day!

Since I couldn't have visitors in my stateroom, my OA friend and I met in her office. This tiny metal cubbyhole with harsh lights, no ventilation, and only a thin divider separating us from two other rooms, became our sanctuary. Sharing the struggle of staying serene in such harsh conditions, we helped each other through homesickness and home-meeting sickness. Before taking this job, I'd aided my abstinence by giving myself treats other than food: baths, walks, flowers, and occasionally new clothes or cosmetics.

The problem was none of these things were available on board. We only had the Big Book, OA literature, our Higher Power, and each other—and it worked! My abstinence was as clean then as it's ever been.

My time on the tender ended suddenly. One hot night, I moved to the upper bunk in hopes of getting some cool air from the fan. At 3 a.m., my phone rang and I, half asleep and forgetting that I'd changed beds, jumped to get it. I fell seven feet onto one-and-a-half-inch plate steel, breaking my right wrist. People heard my screams several decks away.

Twenty-four hours later, with one arm in a cast and my bags packed, I stood on deck wearing a lifejacket, a hard hat, and a harness, waiting to be hoisted off the ship by means of a crane inside one of the huge metal boxes usually used for burning garbage. My OA and AA friends showed up, having slipped away from their duties to say goodbye. We held hands and said the Serenity Prayer. I stepped into the burn box and began my long, painful journey home. The program goodbye was a good start, and I knew that thanks to OA and the worldwide Twelve-Step Fellowship, I would never be alone.

— *San Diego, California USA*

Promising Steps

Shortly after coming to OA almost three years ago, I began to notice a change in my attitudes toward social gatherings, particularly parties. I found myself feeling increasingly uncomfortable at these events and frequently wished I had stayed home. Dinner parties, birthday parties, holiday parties . . . I began to avoid them whenever possible. Unfortunately, this became a problem at home since my wife loves parties and we are frequently invited to them.

Instead of examining my feelings, I justified my stance by rationalizing that refusing to attend parties was "taking care of myself." After all, I thought, parties are just food and alcohol feasts that have no place in my daily eating plan. I was partially correct. When I first gained my abstinence, parties were slippery places for me because of the unlimited food and drink. But as time went on and my recovery progressed, I realized that what made me uncomfortable at parties was my uneasiness with myself and the other guests—not the food.

In the days before I came to OA, I ate and drank my way through parties, thus avoiding having to confront my feelings. Anger, low self-esteem, and fear of people were the underlying causes of my overeating at parties. I often felt less than others, believing I had nothing interesting or important to say. I was also uncomfortable about my 315-pound (143-kg) body, so I preferred not to talk to anyone, convinced they would judge me by my size. These feelings also precipitated my anger, and I actually found myself resenting people who could enjoy themselves.

When I reached a normal weight and remained abstinent, these feelings that had been buried began to resurface. No wonder I didn't like parties—they brought to light some of my most serious defects of character. It was clear that there was work to be done, and the program provided the answer.

I asked HP for help with this problem and resolved to go to the next party with an open mind, willing to confront my discomfort. The first party I attended was tough as my wife was unable to go and I'd always depended on her to keep me company. When I walked in the door, I realized that I didn't know anyone in the room—and all eyes were on me. I was fearful, but I remembered to trust my plan. After the host introduced me to others around the room, I told a few jokes and began to feel more at ease than usual. I saw the spread of food and alcohol but thought, "It's not for me" and chose a diet drink instead. I began getting to know the other guests, moving from person to person. Eventually some people I knew arrived, and I felt even more comfortable; but I realized that it really didn't matter as my Higher Power and I were doing just fine on our own.

One of the promises of the Steps was at work: I found myself intuitively knowing how to handle a situation that used to baffle me. I felt comfortable instead of afraid. Later on we played a party game, (which I'd always hated) and I won! I really had a good time. For the other guests it was probably just another party, but for me it was a breakthrough.

I continue to share my feelings about parties at meetings and with my sponsor because they are a symbol of many other problems I have in my life. My uncomfortable feelings haven't totally disappeared, but they are definitely getting less intense. I don't go to every party that comes along, but I go to many more than before—and I enjoy most of them. My wife has certainly noticed the difference too.

Looking to the program for a solution was the key to my growth in this regard, and it served to strengthen my abstinence and my belief in the OA Twelve-Step way of life.

— *Washington, D.C. USA*

New Way of Living

My husband travels on business about three or four times a year. I used to do some of my worst bingeing while he was out of town. The loneliness and boredom were more than I could bear, and I ate in an effort to fill the emptiness. I felt I deserved to eat in order to comfort myself.

How things have changed! After four years of working an OA program, I now handle my husband's business trips quite differently. The most important change is that I stay abstinent. I don't use his absence as an excuse to binge. When he's gone, I attend extra meetings to remind myself of my disease and to be with people who can hug me and help me feel less lonely. I nurture myself spiritually by working the Steps, by praying, and by attending my church. And I engage in fun, meaningful, and fulfilling activities.

During my husband's most recent absence, I happened upon an idea that may become a regular tradition. I invited three OA friends to my home for a potluck. After an abstinent dinner, we sat in my living room for three hours, talking, sharing, and laughing. It was like having a meeting in my own home.

It's just another example of the many healthy ways I've learned to take care of myself.

— *Chapel Hill, North Carolina USA*

Livin' It Up!

I just returned from a vacation in Orlando, Florida. I acted like any normal, healthy thirteen-year-old, running from one Epcot Center exhibit to another, petting animals at the Busch Gardens petting zoo, and going on rides at Walt Disney World. Higher Power really gave me a chance to enjoy a vacation like a teenager was meant to.

> *Working my program has also given me the power of choice with regard to food.*

The catch? I'm a thirty-three-year-old, recovering compulsive overeater.

As a teenager, I was depressed and unhappy, and I didn't know why. I felt so different from everyone else, and I was sure that no one would like me if they knew the real me (whoever that was). I thought my feelings of ugliness, unacceptability, and separateness were mine alone.

How different my life is because of OA. Now I can share my most intimate thoughts and feelings with another person and know that I am understood, loved, and supported. After eleven years of recovery, seven years of abstinence, and having maintained a 75-pound (34-kg) weight loss, Higher Power is helping me to do things that I never thought I could do for myself. Namely, being able to vacation in Florida for a week and stay abstinent and sane.

I enjoyed the fun, the sun, the entertainment, and the people. I wore shorts and halter tops during the morning and lounged around the pool in a bathing suit all afternoon. Rather than focusing on my problems and my self-centered negativity, I chose instead to focus on the positiveness of the people, places, and things I encountered.

Working my program has also given me the power of choice with regard to food. I used to feel I had to eat my binge foods. I used to believe that food talked to me. I used to think I couldn't say no. Not anymore. Thanks to OA, food is no longer my Higher Power.

— *Boise, Idaho USA*

You Can Take It With You

I am aware of the many gifts of this program as I enjoy my second abstinent summer. I have been relieved of the dread that used to precede the change of seasons and the inevitable wardrobe change that went with it—from comfortably bulky wool to cool, revealing cotton. The dread has been lifted because of the self-acceptance I have been blessed with through the program.

I have also been relieved of the insanity that used to possess me as I prepared for vacations. No more compulsive dieting, obsessive exercising, or frantic shopping for something to wear. Now, I pack only the clothes that fit, abandoning the idea that I could certainly knock off a few pounds while I'm away.

I'm especially careful about packing my program, because without it, my vacation would be a living hell. I make sure to take my literature, my journal, the most recent issue of *Lifeline,* and phone lists.

Probably the most important item I bring is willingness. I must be willing to get down on my knees and turn my will and my life over to my Higher Power first thing every morning, even while on vacation. I must be willing to spend time reading my literature, and to take advantage of leisure time to listen to what HP has to say. I must be willing to look up Overeaters Anonymous in the phone book and make contact with another compulsive overeater.

I recently returned from Virginia Beach after visiting my brother and his wife. I was glad to be with them during the birth of their daughter. While there, I enjoyed walks along the shore and bike rides around the lake. I felt quite comfortable wearing shorts, something I didn't feel worthy of before program.

Actually, my first vacation miracle happened about one year ago, when HP made it possible for me to go to Italy for six weeks, combining my medical training with a vacation. And the gift of abstinence was given to me each day as I turned everything over to God—going to meetings, making new program friends in Milan, and even writing a portion of my Fourth-Step inventory and taking the Fifth Step with a woman who will always be so special to me.

God willing, I hope to return to Italy at the end of this summer. I know that my disease will travel with me, so, gratefully, I'll choose to take my program along too.

— *Philadelphia, Pennsylvania USA*

Abstinence Has No Boundaries

Five years ago, when I was first deciding what my abstinence would be, I followed my own personal guidelines. First, my abstinence had to be livable. To me, that meant I could continue it for a lifetime. Secondly, I had to be able to eat out and still maintain my abstinence. Thirdly, I had to be able to eat abstinently anywhere in the world.

Two years later, and newly at maintenance weight, that third part came in very handy when I learned my husband had received orders to go to Japan for three years. I was so excited about the move. I worried about many things, but oddly enough, abstinence wasn't one of them. I trusted God to be wherever I was.

Our first six weeks in Japan were spent in a hotel until we could find a house. Unable to cook, I ate out three meals a day. With abstinence as my first priority, it was an adventure. At the very least, it was an immediate incentive to learn a little Japanese so I could order or buy the food I needed.

When we moved into our new house, I began making the two-hour trip into Tokyo for OA meetings. By telephone, I began to build the support system that was to sustain me for the next three years. I got two OA pen pals through OA's pen-pal program.* Writing to those OA members became my between-meeting opportunities to strengthen my program.

When traveling, most people have a tendency to want to taste new and exotic foods. I knew that wasn't for me, so I decided I'd find my joy in the people, the country, and the culture. I didn't want my experience spoiled by a return to my illness.

Japanese women, as I was to discover, love to extend hospitality with food, so I was often in the position of having to refuse food. At first, I learned how to say, "I don't eat sugar," in Japanese, but then they were confused when I refused nonsugar foods. I learned to explain my three-meal-a-day abstinence. Sometimes I showed my fat pictures, and explained that I didn't want to return to my former size. Eventually, my friends learned to offer me only coffee or tea.

The most humorous experience in this regard was when one Japanese friend asked me why, after three years of "dieting" (her understanding of my abstinence), did I still look the same? I hadn't considered that it would confuse anyone if I said I was on a diet. She'd probably wondered why I just didn't give up—or at least try a more successful "diet"!

I'm so thankful for my early years in OA when I had heard other members say, "My disease doesn't take a vacation from me, so I can't take a vacation from abstinence." Since I didn't want to lose my abstinence during my time in Japan, I used the tools, worked the Steps, and left the rest to God. Fortunately, I was never afraid to ask my hostesses for help in meeting my abstinence needs. I didn't have to be ashamed of my disease.

I came home a few months ago. I hadn't changed in size, but inside I had grown. I am so grateful I have a portable program, and I can carry it anywhere.

— *Olympia, Washington USA*

*OA's pen-pal program has been discontinued since this article was written.

Flying High With OA

I'm on my way to London, literally, so it seems like a good time to share a bit about how I stay abstinent on the road—and in the air.

Airline seats have become a lot more comfortable since I lost 100 pounds (45 kg), compliments of OA. However, I need to work my OA program just as intensely now as I did when I was first losing that weight six years ago.

Lots of OA meetings are just as essential to me while traveling as when I'm at home because my eating disorder travels with me. In fact, I have a London OA meeting list with me, thanks to one of my sponsees who was there last month.

Food selection while traveling can present some difficulties. Travel schedules, work responsibilities, time differences, and local food availability can make it hard to obtain my preferred foods. Nevertheless, I don't deviate from the basic structure of my food plan. Through many years of trial and error, I have discovered an eating plan that works best for me, and I stick to it. For me, it is much easier to stay abstinent than to get abstinent.

Airlines are quite willing to provide me with a special meal if given advance notice. However, they make mistakes regularly, as they did today. So as a back-up, I carry some abstinent foods on board to eat on such occasions.

Prayer, meditation, reading the Big Book, attending OA meetings, and sending postcards to OA friends back home are just some of the actions I take to stay abstinent on the road. Even transatlantic phone calls are cheaper than bingeing. And if I'm lucky, I'll find someone with whom I can share my program, because working with other compulsive overeaters is the best guarantee I have.

— *Oakland, California USA*

No Games With the Food

I'm a compulsive overeater, abstinent eighteen years by the grace of God and the Twelve Steps. For me, abstinence is freedom from compulsive overeating. It's for the compulsive overeater what sobriety is for the alcoholic. It means I don't take that extra bite—no matter what. It means I eat sanely and reasonably because working the Steps helps me do that. It means my body stays at the same sane weight because I eat right.

I pigged out my first week in OA doing it on my own. Then I got a sponsor who said "first things first . . . put down your fork." She felt strongly that the only Step a person can take while overeating is Step One. After that, she explained, I had to be out of the food to be on the road to recovery.

I chose a plan of eating from the OA pamphlet *Dignity of Choice*. I didn't have a clue what appropriate portions were, so a plan helped me learn. I weighed and measured every meal for three years. I let go of trying to control my food my way and let OA guide me about what and when I should eat. I never tried to keep OA and my disease a secret. It's who I am. If my boyfriend thought it was weird, I didn't need him in my life. If his mother thought it was weird, that was her problem. My problem is I'm a compulsive overeater, and my solution is to go to any lengths to stay abstinent.

During my first year of abstinence, I couldn't go to restaurants often. Once, a basket of bread called out to me from the table. I excused myself from the business luncheon, went to a pay phone and called my sponsor. I told her about the bread's siren voice, said the serenity prayer and returned sane to my meeting. The bread stayed in the basket.

I became abstinent just before the holidays. Prior to visiting my grandmother, my sponsor and I role-played how to say no when my grandmother offered food. I now respect holidays as times to "improve my conscious contact with my Higher Power." This helps me avoid feasting or fasting. I eat the same way every day. I'm a compulsive overeater. I must not play games with food nor take vacations from my plan of eating.

For three years I ate three weighed-and-measured meals with nothing in between and no grains or sugars. We had no cake or champagne at my wedding. We had a potluck dinner, and I brought a sane meal for myself. It was wonderful not to worry about food.

I suffered from morning sickness when pregnant. The doctor told me to eat crackers to combat nausea, but I feared breaking abstinence. This was a turning point. With my sponsor's help, I learned OA doesn't help me eat in a certain way, but helps me eat for my body's health. If I needed grain between meals, I could work the Steps, and my Higher Power would help me.

Sometimes my plan of eating appears rigid and sometimes flexible. I'm willing to accept the limits I need at the moment. My plan of eating started one day at a time, sometimes one minute at a time. It has continued one day at a time for more than 6,400 days. That's a miracle! I pray for lifelong abstinence one day at a time.

— *Anonymous*

Maintaining Long-Term Abstinence

Thanks to my Higher Power's grace, I have been abstinent since 1981. Without abstinence, my relationships with people and with God are much less satisfactory because my focus is on food and dieting. In all circumstances of life, whether vacations or difficulties, I consider my abstinence first.

I keep my program fresh by going to at least two OA meetings a week. As I listen to the pain in a newcomer's voice, I remember my pain. When I see someone return to OA having gained 100 pounds (45 kg) and hear that no other answer was out there, I remember that abstinence is "the easier, softer way." I always speak at meetings, even if only to identify myself. I volunteer to lead meetings because I need to hear my story.

Service keeps me involved. I feel needed by the group and by others. This supports my abstinence.

I always have a sponsor, and I am a sponsor. I commit my food to my sponsor every day at our agreed-upon time. I arrange my schedule so I have an hour each morning to take calls from my sponsees. Talking to my sponsor and my sponsees is like having a meeting each day. They keep me connected.

To serve my group, I have been note taker, key keeper, literature chair and treasurer. I speak to other groups, intergroups or conferences when asked. Service keeps me involved. I feel needed by the group and by others. This supports my abstinence.

I prepare for food situations. If I am going to a restaurant, I call ahead to see if they have the food I need. Sometimes I pack all my food for a weekend retreat so I can focus on my spiritual life. I plan, shop, and cook my food for a week at a time so I will have what I need.

I make the Twelve Steps part of my life. I take Steps One, Two, and Three daily. I have taken Steps Four through Nine at least five times. I have used OA and AA literature to help me. I have participated in a Step-study group and a Big Book study group.

Journaling helps me. I can think more clearly and get in touch with my feelings better when I write. Looking through my past journals helps me see patterns in my life. I can see where my Higher Power has brought good out of what I thought was a bad situation. I realize that everything passes, no matter how terrible I thought it was at the time.

Danger lies in believing the untruths my disease tells me, such as: "Just one won't hurt. I'll eat today and get right back on my food plan. I'll substitute this food and not tell my sponsor. I've measured long enough; surely I know how much to eat by now. I don't have time for meetings. I can do this without a sponsor. These sponsees take up too much time." Without staying connected to OA, to my sponsor and sponsees, to my Higher Power, to all of my program, I can begin to listen to these dangerous lies.

I have attracted others to OA by living my program. Only by weighing and measuring my food in front of others, year after year, was I an attraction. Only by gratitude for my abstinence, by seeing it as freedom from slavery to food and to the ravages of the disease of compulsive overeating, did I attract others.

In dealing with Tradition breaks that might have caused me to leave OA, I have remembered the slogan "Principles over personalities" and talked about my difficulties with my sponsor and with other abstinent members. I have recalled the value of abstinence in my life and realized I cannot be abstinent alone. I have prayed and journaled about the difficulties. As I look back over eighteen and a half years of abstinence, I see that these difficulties have passed.

My abstinence is a gift that I receive anew each day. I am free of the mental and physical slavery to food. I suffer none of the health problems overweight has caused to so many members of my family. I have the benefits of a support group in all my life's trials. I continually learn a new way of life.

— *Austin, Texas USA*

Joint Effort

I've been thinking a lot about abstinence and trigger foods—not because I'm struggling, but because I'm not struggling. I am one of those fortunate souls who found abstinence immediately and never lost it. I have had minor slips and slides, of course, but nothing serious. Even during those slips, I've never eaten any of my trigger foods. Why am I able to do this easily while others struggle so much?

I figured out that handing it over to HP was only part of it. Asking HP to take it from me and then waiting for the urge to leave didn't work. I did that for years before coming to OA. The way I think about abstinence is what finally did it for me, and still does.

I came to OA to find sanity. I didn't care about weight loss (although I was overweight). I was crazy and couldn't stand it anymore. So right from the start my focus was on that, not on the food. I understood that trigger foods interfere with sanity and peace because they create cravings I have to struggle to resist. Without those foods, the cravings are not there. Occasionally they rear their heads, but they're weak and disappear almost immediately. So having "a little hit" occasionally wouldn't be a treat; it would be a struggle. To say it's not worth it is a huge understatement. I won't consider it, period.

Do I feel deprived? No! My trigger foods (sweets) are not food; they are simply things I don't eat, so they don't call to me. They're a nonissue.

Not eating between meals is another tool in my food plan I hold on to. Three meals, one snack, no sweets, that's it. No counting, measuring, weighing, or focusing on the food; I focus on other things, and I have a life I can live now. I don't have to squeeze it in between bites of food, and I don't use food as an excuse to not live my life. I have lots of time now to do things and more room in my head to think about things other than food.

I'm not telling you this to brag, my friends. I am humble. My part in this only works because I ask God daily to lift the compulsion from me, and he does. I do my footwork and he does the rest.

I hear so much anguish around food and abstinence in my group.

Letting go of my food meant not trying to control it through my old dieting. Letting go gave me the freedom to be abstinent. Letting go of control didn't send it out of control, only out of my control. HP is controlling it all nicely and is much better at it than I could ever be. I feel peaceful, calm, and not afraid anymore, which is a much more significant gift than the weight loss I've experienced. That is a nice side effect, but it doesn't come close to the changes inside!

— *Toronto, Ontario Canada*

New Day, New Life

When I wake up in the morning, I give thanks for the gifts of this day and my life.

The new day is full of possibilities, and one possibility is to live abstinently. I am a compulsive overeater who for many years didn't know such a possibility existed. Now I see that abstinence itself is a gift, and every day I can consciously choose to accept or reject this gift. OA defines abstinence as the act of refraining from compulsive overeating, but for me it begins with the act of choosing to accept the gift.

> *The new day is full of possibilities, and one possibility is to live abstinently.*

I relinquish all thoughts of "having to abstain," just as I relinquish results and focus instead on doing the next right thing.

My job is to cherish the gift and take good care of it. To do this, I need to make a plan of eating, use the other tools of recovery and work the Twelve Steps. In practical terms, Step Eleven is most important for me. I take a few moments before each meal to express my gratitude for this day, this life, and this food I am about to eat. (As I write this, I realize it is important to do this *whenever* I'm about to put something in my mouth.) Let it nourish my body, mind, and spirit. I do this silently, after closing my eyes for a few seconds.

I recently witnessed an animated discussion of food plans, and afterward someone in a wistful tone asked to hear more about the role of spirituality in abstinence. For me, nothing is more important to my abstinence than doing my spiritual push-ups so I may remain spiritually fit. I accept the gift and cherish it for 24 hours. Then I go to sleep having lived abstinently for one more day.

I know this may sound foreign to newcomers. Many newcomers, myself included, come to OA and express something like "I really, really want to gain control of my eating."

Newcomers want to know how to begin, where to start, what to do, and which food plan to follow. When I work with newcomers, I make sure they tell me their diet story. I want them to remind themselves what they've done in the past to try to control their compulsive overeating.

When they've finished, I tell them my secret: despite my many years of recovery, I have no control over my compulsive overeating. Instead, I admit my powerlessness as expressed in Step One. I explain that by admitting powerlessness, I have eleven other Steps that offer something much more powerful than control. These Steps offer a way of life that one day at a time frees me from addiction and affords me a life of serenity, peace, and physical well-being.

If that's not a gift, I don't know what is.

One of the promises of this program is that we will have a new way of acting on life, rather than reacting to it. My new way of acting includes everything I've shared in this writing. For me, abstinence is not a single act, but rather is the result of taking many other small "next right actions." This results in the gift of abstinence that is offered in the waking moments of each new day. Thinking about it this way is an immense help to me.

— *Anonymous*

Thanksgiving Anniversary

I came to OA twenty-three years ago, and I've always found it relevant that I entered program just before the much-abused holiday of Thanksgiving. My relationship to Thanksgiving was typical: I stuffed myself until I was miserable, loaded up on carbs and desserts, and felt sick the rest of the day.

Before my first meeting, I weighed 340 pounds (154 kg). I was a physician, and my own doctor had told me I wouldn't be able to work much longer if I didn't lose weight. I had frequent, severe chest pain that started when my dangerously high blood pressure had been brought down with medication to acceptable levels.

> *My recovery has been slow but steady, and abstinence has meant different things at different times.*

The arthritis in my hips, back, and legs was so bad I could hardly get out of bed. I was clinically depressed and had been since childhood. I was the product of a fundamentalist religious upbringing with a harsh, punitive God. Suicide was always in the back of my mind as a viable option, and I had a plan. I was 43 years old, married, and had two beautiful little girls, but I could see no way out.

I am now sixty-seven and count my life a miracle. My recovery has been slow but steady, and abstinence has meant different things at different times. My Higher Power has taught me about nourishment and exercise—I'm a slow learner.

I was in program ten years before I finally admitted I had to give up a major binge food. I was in program sixteen years before I could consistently work toward giving up sugar and white flour. This was necessary before I could have surgery so I could heal well and not have wound infections (which I had had many years before while eating those substances).

I now live in abstinence, which consists of no chocolate, wheat, or sugar and focuses on small portions of healthy foods. I've had a great deal of help from my Higher Power and my OA sisters and brothers.

The only times I stopped walking the path occurred when I stopped attending meetings. I can use all the other tools, but if I don't attend meetings it's as though I am not "plugged in," and I relapse in a bad way. Both times when I stopped attending meetings, I regained 50 to 60 pounds (23 to 27 kg) or more.

I have no idea how high my weight got because my medical center did not have scales that could weigh me. Sanity and abstinence came back only after I returned to meetings.

I'm about to retire from my regular employment so my wife and I can travel. At this point I am sustaining a 166-pound (76-kg) weight loss. I don't have high blood pressure and have not had chest pain in years. I still have some arthritis, but take medicine for it only occasionally. I receive medical help for the things I need, but they do not include diabetes, heart disease, or high blood pressure, diseases I was heading toward in my forties. That is why I keep coming back!

— *Anonymous*

Pregnancy and Recovery

I am three weeks from the due date of my first child. I have abstained from eating compulsively one day at a time for more than six years, including the last nine months. My pregnancy has gone like the rest of my recovery, with prayer, meetings, and much help and by putting my relationship with my Higher Power first.

I am living a rich, full, wonderful, abstinent life, one day at a time. The mechanics of maintaining abstinence in pregnancy were simple. At my first prenatal visit, the doctor told me to trust my

> *I needed direction because I couldn't rely on my own judgment or appetite.*

body and eat healthy food in moderation as my appetite dictated. I explained that I have followed a structured way of eating for several years, and I wasn't sure how to alter it for pregnancy.

I received a referral to a nutritionist. I prayed for guidance before visiting her. I also prayed to surrender any attempt to control my food or plan of eating and to trust the nutritionist. I needed direction because I couldn't rely on my own judgment or appetite. Doing that had left me defeated, self-hating, and unhealthy when I walked through the doors of my first OA meeting seven and a half years ago.

I gave the nutritionist a synopsis of my story, focusing on my need for explicit directions to follow during my pregnancy so I could be healthy and sane to take care of the baby and myself. She gave me a structured food plan that has served me well for the last seven months.

The most challenging aspects of my pregnancy have been spiritual and emotional. I have had to practice turning over my body, life, fears, and unborn baby to God every day. I have especially had to practice surrendering my changing figure and my fear in the early stages of pregnancy that people would think I was overeating. Refraining from immediately telling everyone, "I'm not in relapse; I'm pregnant" was a good exercise in humility. Instead, I prayed to keep my mouth shut.

Now that I'm in the final weeks of pregnancy, fears about my ability to give birth and be a good mother are bothering me. I find it imperative to surrender daily to my Higher Power and to continue working the Twelve Steps, sponsoring and trying to get out of myself and into helping others. I have faith my baby and I will be well taken care of through labor, birth, and the rest of our lives together.

As long as I continue to abstain from eating compulsively, reach out to other members of Overeaters Anonymous, and practice the Twelve Steps and Twelve Traditions, I will receive the help I need and the "life beyond my wildest dreams" OA promised at my first meeting. The last nine months have been among the best of my recovery. The credit goes to OA, God, and abstinence.

— *Port Angeles, Washington USA*

CHAPTER SEVEN

How Abstinence Changes with Time and Experience

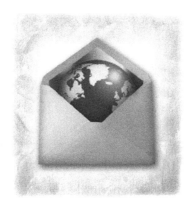

Still Works

I became abstinent almost six years ago at age 62. My abstinence has not been a struggle, but the aging process comes with its own struggles. Abstinence has enhanced my ability to live through those struggles, and to have more energy and a light heart.

> *Food is no longer my god—it's my nourishment.*

I hope aging in OA, attending meetings, and sponsoring enhance the quality of the OA program and Fellowship. The focus must be on the solution—not the problem. We have the same problem, but we know the solution: a Power greater than ourselves. The Big Book gives precise directions on how to find this power: "If I focus on a problem, the problem increases; if I focus on the answer, the answer increases" (*Alcoholics Anonymous*, 4th ed., p. 419).

When I returned to OA seven years ago, I was on one of my diets. I white-knuckled it for some months before surrendering and getting a sponsor who had what I wanted. I slowly managed to achieve a goal weight and have maintained my weight within a five-pound (2-kg) range. I do this by weighing myself once a month and adjusting my food intake accordingly. My exercise is consistent. My food plan enables me to choose proper amounts of nontrigger foods. My footwork is to follow it, and I do.

As I age and my body changes, I will continue to do what I have always done, and I will get the same wonderful results. I will adjust my food to maintain a healthy weight.

Aging abstinently is a gift I cherish. Abstinence has led me back to my Higher Power. Food is no longer my god—it's my nourishment.

— *Croton-on-Hudson, New York USA*

Most Important Thing

I am approaching one year of first-time abstinence in this OA program. What a difference a year can make! I don't want to talk about the cessation of food hangovers and comas or relief from the desire to numb out in fast food—bags and boxes of junk. For these changes I have extraordinary gratitude, but I want to talk about where I am today.

Within my first couple of program months, my food was clean ninety-seven percent of the time. I shed the final 15 pounds (7 kg) that had been plaguing me. By my fifth month, I was 2 pounds (1 kg) under my goal weight. What joy! What cause for celebration! But in the grand scheme of things, it didn't bring me what I thought it would.

When I was fourteen years old, I thought my life would begin when I reached my goal weight. Men would line up, my career would take off, and I'd have a booming social life. My outer world would finally live up to my ideal. More than a decade later, I reached that goal weight. But would it surprise you to hear that none of my "if/then" scenarios happened?

The best gift from being at goal weight is the serenity, joy and comfort I feel in my body. I can wear anything and feel great in my skin. At the time I achieved goal weight, I was a part-time exercise instructor. I was go-go-go four to five days a week, taking and teaching many classes.

I was also running around town going on auditions and attending one to two (sometimes three) meetings a day. I was super active, so of course I reached goal weight and beyond in a short time.

Since that time in program, my schedule has undergone a dramatic shift. Instead of teaching fitness classes, I work a sedentary job forty hours a week. Instead of being involved in physical activity four to five days a week, I am lucky if I have the energy and time to make it to two fitness classes. I also have to balance meetings in two programs. Clothes that used to fit me loosely four months ago aren't so loose these days. But the miracle is my clothes still fit.

Does this mean I should throw my program away or give up and stuff my face in some food to feel better? Back when I was full into the disease, I used weight gain as an excuse to eat to "feel better."

For today I have another solution. First I must admit I am powerless over what I look like and it's just none of my daggone business. I am abstinent. By not compulsively overeating, I'm choosing not to add insult to injury. I'll be frank: I don't feel my sexiest right now. I feel bigger, and sometimes I look in the mirror and yearn for my sub-goal-weight body back. But my sponsor ingrained in me from the get-go to ask myself how I can be kind, loving, and gentle to myself, especially when I feel the most unbalanced.

So for today I focus on what makes me feel good and allows me to take care of myself. This morning that was waking up early to do my laundry and clean my home. These activities allow me to give myself the gift of clean clothes and a refreshed home.

What works for me is doing physical activity three to four times a week. I trust I will resume this activity soon, but I am entrusting the details to my Higher Power. I am holding onto the faith that I will feel amazing in my body again and the little extra weight I've put on since my schedule change will take care of itself.

Until that day (and even after it), I choose to focus on my connection with my Higher Power, because that's what this program is about: maintaining the constant contact that relieves the compulsion to act out with unhealthy food behaviors.

I'm not thrilled with how my clothes fit now, but for today I am abstinent. That is the most important thing.

— *Southern California USA*

Blessed Event

Having been blessed with abstinence and physical recovery, being pregnant made me view my program in an entirely new way.

Out went my three-meals-a-day abstinence. Being blighted with nausea for three months made me ask God for the willingness to be more flexible with my food. My abstinence changed each day as my pregnancy progressed. It felt comfortable because my food was being controlled by God.

Back came the scale into my life. My own had been thrown out long ago. Now doctors and midwives needed to monitor my weight gain. At first this terrified me, bringing back feelings and memories associated with diet clubs. But I shared my fears honestly with my sponsor, and, after the first weigh-in, the fears dissolved.

Once more I had to contend with an expanding waistline. I had trouble separating my feelings about what a swelling stomach meant in the past from what it means during pregnancy. All those old emotions of guilt and remorse after a binge needed to be dealt with promptly.

The discomfort of tight waistbands meant the baby was getting bigger, not me! But switching to elasticized pants and baggy tops and putting "normal" clothes away for the future made me think of my pre-OA days. I had to remind myself that I live each day in recovery lovingly supported by OA friends. This expansion in my body meant a new life—for me as well as the baby.

I gave birth to a beautiful baby daughter. In God's timing, the gift of physical recovery returned as though it had never disappeared. Maybe to God it had been there all along.

— *Nottingham, England*

Opening Windows

Last summer we started renovating our big, old house. I'd been in OA for three years, had lost 80 pounds (36 kg), and was enjoying a clean abstinence, one day at a time.

I was excited about getting a new kitchen and bathroom. The old ones were dark and cramped, and I longed to knock down the old walls, put in lots of beautiful new windows, and bring in some sunshine and fresh air.

During the construction I struggled with my eating. It was hard to stay abstinent, I rationalized, because my kitchen was all torn up, and I couldn't cook properly. The stress of the expense of the project and the unexpected delays and complications made it hard for me to meditate and exercise.

When it was completed, the house was beautiful, and I was 20 pounds (9 kg) heavier and desperate to find a way back to the serenity I had once enjoyed.

As I struggled, my Higher Power reminded me of the windows I had needed in my home. I realized that I need to open windows, one day at a time, to work my OA program as well.

When I call my sponsor, it feels as if I've opened a window and let in the fresh morning air. When I take time to read OA literature and meditate, the warm sunshine of understanding shines on my face.

Whenever I go to a meeting, I feel like I'm opening a window that lets me see where I'm going and where I've been.

I used to feel that "working my program" was indeed work. But now it's as easy to me as opening windows—and how much joy, strength, and comfort I get from living with sunshine and fresh air! I realize that I want to use the tools of the program—my beautiful windows—every day.

— *Minneapolis, Minnesota USA*

Perfection Not Required

One night I walked away from the dinner table discouraged, my body sluggish from too much food, and my heart lonely. I'd been abstinent for three and a half years, lost more than 100 pounds (45 kg), and hadn't felt this way since before I joined OA.

I wasn't eating my binge foods or eating between meals. But the meals were becoming too big. Why? I realized that nearly six weeks had passed since I'd attended a meeting. And I remembered many phone calls from concerned OA friends that I'd failed to return. I was still reading my literature and writing in my journal every day, but apparently this wasn't enough.

At first I blamed my increased appetite on a new medication. But I had to admit this was only an excuse. I'd been using a recurring illness to isolate myself, and that was leading me back to my old friend and enemy, food.

Dealing with the illness was difficult enough; now I was slipping back into old habits. Did I have the strength to change? Writing in my journal helped me realize that I didn't need strength—what I needed was the willingness to admit my powerlessness, ask for help, and begin anew.

I asked my Higher Power to help me. I committed to attending at least one meeting a week. I began making phone calls. I wrote down my food every day (something I never had to do before) and continued to read and write. Every morning, I turned my will over to my Higher Power, and every evening I went to bed grateful for another good program day.

As I write this, a month has passed. It's now spring. The air is crisp and clear, the leaves are budding anew, and so is my life. My health is only slightly better, but once again I feel connected. I'm going to meetings, using the phone, and staying abstinent. And, best of all, I'm grateful to have a program that allows me to recover even when I'm less than perfect.

— *Quincy, Massachusetts USA*

Relapse Happens

I used to hear, "Relapse is a part of recovery," and discount it because I thought it meant that everyone is going to relapse sooner or later. I learned that it's a paraphrase for "Relapse happens."

Why do people relapse? Is relapse avoidable? Is it inevitable? These questions are all so meaningless because the only thing that matters is that relapse does happen. Debate over the legitimacy of relapse only serves to shame us and—as we all know—shame never motivated

It was when I finally accepted that I was in relapse that I felt my HP's presence again.

any of us to do anything but hide and eat. We need acceptance instead of debate.

I thought relapse would never happen to me. I was working the Steps, measuring my food, calling my sponsor—what could go wrong? When I hit goal weight I started to slip. I hung on to my old ideas about abstinence, program, and relapse until I choked the very life out of them, only letting on at meetings that I was having "a little trouble with my food," I wondered where my Higher Power was. It was when I finally accepted that I was in relapse that I felt my HP's presence again. I felt a hand on my shoulder and the beginning of the most spiritual journey in my recovery. I learned that God's love is absolutely unconditional. No matter what I've done, where I'm at, or what I'm putting in my mouth, my HP is right there letting me know that I'm accepted and I must accept myself (and others) in the same way. My Higher Power is always in the present moment. Since I couldn't accept that I was in relapse, I wasn't living in the present and couldn't find my Higher Power. I got back in touch with the reality of the moment, and I learned to value my abstinence for the miracle that it really is.

Could I have avoided relapse? I don't know. But I don't regret it. It taught me that weighing and measuring is not the only way to be abstinent, that it's not true that only abstinent people have something of value to say, and that arrogance is an immediate food-trigger for me. The experience solidified my trust in HP's presence in good times and bad, made me a humbler, gentler person, and got me back in touch with the meaning of "fellow sufferers." It also made me a more seasoned sponsor. The way to sponsor people in relapse is to give them exactly what my HP gave me, to let them know that I accept them unconditionally—without judgment—and encourage them to keep coming back.

— *Schenectady, New York USA*

Progress Report

When I first came into OA more than thirteen years ago, one of the first things my sponsor asked me to do was to write out a history of my weight gains and losses in order to get a clear picture of the nature of my disease. Now, after so many years in OA, I find it useful to review all the different ways I've tried to work this program.

At my first OA meeting I was given a food plan. Abstinence was clearly defined as following this food plan without exception, and committing my food every day to a sponsor. It was very easy to know when I broke my abstinence: An extra lettuce leaf meant that I had to restart the abstinence count from zero. A lot of things depended on clean abstinence back then, such as the right to be a sponsor, which required twenty-one days of back-to-back abstinence.

It was all made very clear, but nonetheless I could never stay abstinent for more than twelve days in a row. Although learning that I had a disease and was not just weak-willed lightened my load, I still felt like a failure because I could never achieve longterm abstinence. Furthermore, I felt like a fraud because I never talked about my problems. But, in spite of it all, I gave service, including sponsoring. But, oh, how I struggled with abstinence.

Then a new spirit entered OA. It became accepted that some members needed to work a spiritual program in order to become abstinent; that abstinence was a result of spiritual progress.

What an enormous relief! I worked very hard on the Steps, doing a thorough Fourth-Step inventory, and I really tackled my character defects. I wasn't gaining any weight; in fact, I was a little bit thinner. More importantly, I no longer felt guilt nor dishonesty. This was liberating.

I'm grateful for this period in my OA life because it succeeded in eliminating the guilt I was still carrying about my compulsive overeating. But even then long-term abstinence did not appear. Furthermore, I stopped dealing with the food altogether. I no longer worried about what I was eating or how. I did more than give up the scale and the measuring cup—I gave up abstinence as a goal.

During this period of time I was diagnosed as an active diabetic who had to stay on a very careful diet in order to prevent long-term complications. The dietitian gave me a food plan to follow, but I didn't: I just couldn't somehow, perhaps because I didn't have the tools to handle food restrictions as a goal. Or perhaps I believed that it would be all right if I just worked my program, came to meetings, did service, and turned the problem over to my Higher Power.

Two years ago my diabetes worsened, and the dreaded complications became evident. My way may have given me emotional and spiritual progress, but my eating habits were killing me. I didn't know what to do.

Finally I confided in a close OA friend, a nurse, and said I needed help. The experts she sent me to all said that I had to change my eating habits. I really tried, but still I felt it would all work out if I just went to a lot of meetings and did a lot of service.

Nothing much changed. My life was out of control, my food was out of control, and I was slowly killing myself—all the while going to five meetings a week and working my program as hard as I could.

Five months ago, I had a spiritual awakening of the kind I'd always dreamed about. Sitting in my room feeling that I had to choose between life and death (and an ugly death at that), I chose life.

The meaning of that decision became immediately apparent. It meant I had to declare complete bankruptcy and to surrender totally. In this case, surrender clearly meant doing anything and everything I was told to do by my doctor, my dietitian, my sponsor, and the OA literature—everything, without selection, and without exception.

The dietitian told me what to eat and how often, and to follow that plan exactly. It is my abstinence, and it is the most important thing in my life without exception. My doctor tells me what to do and I do it, without complaining. The program tells me that I must be honest and not hide anything, even the smallest issue, and so I'm doing that.

For the first time in more than thirteen years in OA, I am experiencing long-term, continuous abstinence. For the most part the compulsion to overeat has been lifted, and for this I am very grateful.

It is not because I am a diabetic that I can be abstinent—I couldn't be abstinent for years in spite of the fact that I knew what the diabetes was doing to me. I am abstinent today because I have a program that gives priority to abstinence. I take care of the food and the rest just happens.

My program is not the same one I worked thirteen years ago. Now I know that the spiritual and emotional growth I've experienced in OA is part of the entire recovery process. And now there's no guilt associated with less than one 100 percent perfect adherence to a food plan—I just keep trying to make progress.

— *Israel*

An Amazing, Abstinent Life

I spent years trying to control my weight and my eating. Attempts to diet only led me to bingeing. I knew the Steps worked because I was in another Twelve-Step program, so I believed OA would be the answer. Unfortunately, I couldn't find a strong OA meeting in my area that worked for me.

Alone, my progress was slow and faltering. Abstinence eluded me until I realized I had to give up my binge foods entirely, just as the alcoholic must give up alcohol entirely. Like the alcoholic who stops eating normally and wants only alcohol, I only wanted sweets and had to force myself to eat "real" food. It took me two tries to give up sugar, and I went through withdrawal for three days. After that the cravings began to disappear. Abstaining from sweets made me a much saner person and stabilized my weight to a large degree. Until then, I had been gaining weight steadily until I reached my

> *Like the alcoholic who stops eating normally and wants only alcohol, I only wanted sweets and had to force myself to eat "real" food.*

high of 180 pounds (82 kg). I still overate healthy foods and was unable to find a solution to that problem until I finally found strong OA meetings.

In 1990 I returned to OA in desperation. I went to many different meetings until I found a location with strong, three-fold recovery. Through that meeting and the OA *Abstinence* book, I found a plan of eating that worked for me. I eat three moderate meals a day and healthy snacks if necessary. I avoid problem eating behaviors, such as second helpings and eating on the run. I do not eat sweets.

Becoming abstinent from all problem foods wasn't as clear-cut as giving up sweets. Slowly I gained more serenity, lost more weight, and grew in my recovery. Periods of total abstinence grew longer, and through them I was able to glimpse how free and happy life can be without compulsive overeating.

Today I am at a healthy weight and wear a size nine. My clothes fit, and I usually feel good about my appearance. I am mostly free of that overwhelming obsession to eat. The obsession returns at times, but it passes if I am abstinent.

I have worked the Steps to the best of my ability and have done several Fourth Steps. The Steps and slogans are part of my daily life. Sometimes I get off track, but circumstances and my Higher Power lead me back to where I need to be. I go to several meetings a week and read literature every day at breakfast. I use my sponsor and keep in touch with my Higher Power many times each day.

My life has changed greatly since I came to OA. I had a son, left an unhealthy fifteen-year marriage, bought a house, had health problems, traveled all over the country on my motorcycle, and developed some measure of self-esteem and confidence. I am not yet the person I want to be, but I am much better than I was. I see progress through every challenge I face. The most difficult challenge has been to feel my emotions without numbing myself and escaping to food. I am forty years old, and amazing things continue to happen to me. As long as I am abstinent, I am free to experience life and its infinite possibilities.

— *Middletown, New York USA*

The Relief of Honesty

I've been in OA five years, became abstinent by my Higher Power's grace, and worked what I thought was an honest program. I used the tools as best I could and did the footwork. However, this year a restless feeling crept in that I couldn't put my finger on. My food plan changed as I tried to deal with a recurring skin condition; food changes can still throw me off course. I talked with my sponsor and HP and committed to trying this new way of eating.

After three months, my skin showed insignificant changes. Food was not the problem! This unsettled me. Didn't HP know how hard I had worked to eliminate

> *I had been playing games with my food and eating behaviors, and it was robbing me of serenity and spiritual peacefulness.*

and substitute food types? Didn't he understand it had to fix the condition?

For the next couple of months I began to reintroduce foods and regain balance within my food plan. But the obsession kept living with me. I had experienced incredible freedom from the obsession for much of my time in OA, so to be living with it again was uncomfortable and scary. I often felt on the brink of relapse and lived in fear, which I didn't know how to escape.

Then HP showed me how to move forward with humility and spirituality. One morning during my quiet time, I knew I had to admit I had broken my abstinence. I had had no dairy-hopping binges, no hiding or stealing of food; in fact, no specific moment brought me to this realization. But as God spoke to me, I recalled how often I had used my correction pen on my food plan. I have always written down my food plan, but now I saw how shrewd I had become at manipulating, deleting, and adding food to suit my whims. I justified this by telling myself I was not eating compulsively and the eating always ended, so it couldn't be compulsive eating, could it? I had been playing games with my food and eating behaviors, and it was robbing me of serenity and spiritual peacefulness. My disease was active in its own way, and I could not justify or excuse my behaviors just because I wasn't in full-blown bingeing relapse.

I felt like my spirit's light bulb had been switched on! I cannot explain the unbelievable liberation I felt. I raced inside to ring my sponsor. Hearing myself say, "I have broken my abstinence" was freeing. I rang my sponsees and told them. I could hardly wait to tell the group. Never in my OA life did I think I would feel so excited about breaking my abstinence!

This program requires nothing less than rigorous honesty. God has returned my calm spirit. My food and associated behaviors feel clean, and the obsession is not there for today. I am restored to sanity.

OA delivers miracles. I'm sad to think I need to build the length of abstinence to offer myself once more for particular service positions, but God is showing me that service begins with me, here, now. I must continue daily contact with others in OA. I must put my bottom on a meeting seat, share honestly, and give without thought of getting. Spiritual freedom is a gift too precious to put at risk.

— *New Zealand*

No Person, Place, or Thing

I'm grateful for twenty-five years of abstinence—a miracle indeed. When I came to OA in 1980, I couldn't even wait fifteen minutes before eating.

What do I mean when I say, "I am abstinent?" Abstinence means I am free from compulsive overeating and from eating certain foods. When I came to OA, other members suggested I choose a food plan from the *Dignity of Choice* brochure. I chose a simple one and have eaten that way ever since. It's balanced, reasonable,

> *I learned no food plan is better than another, and the best provides what my body needs.*

and healthy, but I've had to change it a few times. I've had two children while in program. I remember the day my doctor said I needed to snack on crackers between meals to stop my pregnancy queasiness. I was scared. I had eaten no grains for three years, and I'd been weighing and measuring my foods; it was working. I'd lost 30 pounds (14 kg) and had been stable for two and a half years.

I learned no food plan is better than another, and the best provides what my body needs. When I ate those first four crackers, I was on the phone with my sponsor to be sure I wasn't being dishonest or deceitful. I remember the wonderful feeling that my Higher Power would help me eat in whatever way I needed and that I could change my plan if that were the next right thing.

The next big change came when I moved to rural Africa. I had no phone or electricity and was not near regular shopping facilities. I had to let go of my scale, trusting my Higher Power.

I have always been willing to measure if I needed to. I also "count" my food, often keeping meals simple by having one or two of certain foods. After the birth of each child, I added a bit to my regular meal plan because I no longer needed the crackers. When I stopped nursing, I went back to my original plan. Now, twenty-five years later, I'm fifty years old and not running around as much. I've let go of a bit of breakfast protein; it seems to work fine.

Abstinence is still the most important thing in my life without exception. I don't have food cravings for years at a time—what a miracle! I've had a slip every four or five years, and each time I was wrapped up in a resentment or fear. I would immediately move to a Tenth-Step inventory and contact my sponsor. That would end it.

Today no person, place, thing, or situation presents me with a good reason to overeat—a good reason to do a Tenth Step! As long as I take daily inventory, work to stay in conscious contact with my Higher Power, and carry the message to newcomers, abstinence continues to be a gift for which I am grateful.

I'm also grateful for my home meeting, where others are abstinent and walking the road of happy destiny.

— *Rowville, Australia*

CHAPTER EIGHT

What Abstinence Has Taught Me

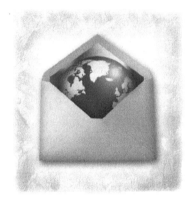

Great Equalizer

Somewhere, sometime, I received a little reminder of meeting topics that listed "equality" as a Traditions topic. Traditions Eleven and Twelve, which deal with anonymity, and Step Seven, which deals with humility, come to mind when I think of equality as a topic (and perhaps Tradition Two).

I've struggled with feeling superior because I have been blessed with long-term abstinence. I see myself as surrendered to a method of staying abstinent. A tendency to feel superior about methods is a frequent factor in OA controversies, and we continue to struggle to overcome or fend off that tendency. Vigilance is required of me to realize and remember that surrender is the gift of a power greater than myself—a power that *is*, even when I don't like it that much.

Feeling "big of myself" is a pitfall of success in physical recovery, and a sense of equality may be as elusive as abstinence. The great equalizer is need. As *Our Invitation to You* says, "It is weakness, not strength, that binds us to each other." Somehow, beyond my understanding and control, it has worked. I am a recipient of mercy that undoes internal opposition. I am needy of this grace and of the recognition that, in our desperate need for this grace (this merciful bringing about of willingness), we are all equal.

I've wondered of late whether I'm sincere enough about my spiritual life. A sponsor might tell me, "Forget the question. You're not sincere enough. Ask your HP to work inside of you, to supply the sincerity that isn't yours."

Recognizing my great need of this grace is necessary for a spirit of equality.

— *Anonymous*

Life After Loss

> *If I look deep enough, even on my worst days I can be thankful for much.*

Finding abstinence and reaching my goal weight are real miracles in my life. Letting go of the extra weight and accepting abstinence with deep gratitude have taken me years to accomplish. In the process I have let go of 50 pounds (23 kg).

I hid behind the fortress of my extra weight. Life had delivered devastating blows, and I thought food was my comfort. In 1984 my husband and I lost two of our five sons. Jody was manic-depressive. Despite our efforts, his demons took over, and he ended his life. He had never recovered from serving as a medic in the Vietnam War. Then two men looking for money attacked our son, Paul. Someone found his body lying by a mountain stream.

These events devastated our family. My husband, our remaining sons, and I left the area and began the long process of rebuilding our lives. My husband drew on years of recovery in AA. I helped establish the first OA meeting in our mountain town. I knew I had to work my OA program and felt in my heart that if God really existed, he had forgotten us.

Fifty pounds (23 kg) later, I was desperate to lose the weight. I kept going to meetings, but the essence of program eluded me. I had hoped I might be one of the lucky ones who somehow magically lost the extra pounds.

Many changes have happened since 1984. Our three sons have done well. Our youngest received his doctorate in neuropsychology. Their progress awes me. Two years ago, doctors diagnosed my husband of forty-six years with leukemia. We have used alternative therapies, and his progress amazes the doctors.

We take life a day at a time. As long as I maintain an "attitude of gratitude," my weight remains low and my heart sings with all I have been given. We often care for our two little grandchildren; I love it!

I have begun a writing career. I have no idea how things will go, but it's the journey and the sharing of what I've learned with those interested that keep me involved. At the close of each day, I write in my journal about what I am grateful for that day. If I really look deep enough, even on my worst days I can be thankful for much. God is doing for me what I am powerless to do for myself.

— *Boulder City, Nevada USA*

Thursday Night Friends

My dad learned he had cancer with no more than six months to live. That's not much time for anyone, especially for a man of forty-six with two small grandchildren. He would not see their birthdays, first days at school, Christmas programs or quality participation at his son's upcoming wedding. The future looked bleak.

With my faith in question and family structure threatened, I had OA beside me during one of the worst periods of my life. OA members called when I needed the understanding voice of a friend, and unconditional love and help to stand when I thought I couldn't. They gave me strength to face each day and find humor in the oddest, most stressful situations.

> *It takes a person to get abstinent, a Higher Power to guide that person, and a group to support that abstinence.*

As I watched my beloved dad fade, my heart broke. I had only six months of abstinence and swore I wouldn't give it up for food. I was determined to feel every pain-filled moment and would not give up on myself as I had done my whole life. Food wouldn't give my dad a miracle or bring him back when it was over. I clung to that realization as my lifeline (even now when grief gets tough, it is my lifeline to sanity). For the first time, I felt every emotion without the comfort of food. The feelings were intense, but I'm glad I felt them.

My sponsor was incredible. Never did she say I shouldn't feel, think or act a certain way. She let me rage like a lion, howl like a wolf, cry like a baby and say what was on my mind, right or wrong, never criticizing. She gave unconditional love and a refuge when I was lost. She listened when no one else would or knew how, knowing she couldn't fix the problem and never suggesting an answer because we knew there was none. Listening was the best gift she could have given. Others wanted to fix or avoid the situation; that doesn't make it go away.

On the day Dad died, I attended my Thursday-night OA meeting; I had nowhere else to go. I felt like eating, and I wanted to be where others understood me. With no tears and numb with grief, I announced Dad had died. My sponsor cried for me. No one had ever done that. She didn't know my dad; she cried because she cared for me. My group surrounded me with more support than I thought possible.

To keep my anonymity, the group sent a basket of flowers to the wake signed, "From your Thursday-night friends." I thought it was from Dad's friends. Mom observed that Dad always came home at night; who could these friends be? I replied, "He must have done something. Those flowers are beautiful." My husband took one look and said, "These are *your* Thursday-night friends." I felt confused, trying to think of what I did on Thursday nights that could inspire such a lovely basket. Then it hit me! I broke into a huge smile, and my heart filled with warmth.

Until then I hadn't realized how much family my OA family is. Every group member attended that wake. Their presence helped me through my life's toughest day. I thank God for each of them. Without them, I would not have achieved over a year's worth of abstinence and a 55-pound (25-kg) weight loss. It takes a person to get abstinent, a Higher Power to guide that person, and a group to support that abstinence.

— *Amboy, Minnesota USA*

Plugged Into Recovery

February 10, 1964, is a date I will never forget. It was my first OA meeting. I was fifty-eight, I weighed around 270 pounds (122 kg), and I was still searching for the magic diet that would do what no other had.

I stormed out of the meeting because what I was hearing was "an insult to my intelligence."

I went to another meeting the very next night. I identified with the speaker and decided to give it a chance. OA was on probation.

At this second meeting I was introduced to the "gray sheet." I got a scale and a cup as had been suggested, and I was ready for business. I was told that I couldn't trust my judgment, and that it would help if I called my food in to someone every day, making the commitment to eat exactly what was measured out. The result would be nirvana!

After twenty-two years of abstinence, my weighing and measuring days are a long way behind me. Recently I heard someone share that she's been in the program for twenty-one years and still calls in her food. To each her own, is something I've learned through twenty-nine years in the program. I'd like to share some other things recovery has taught me.

- Be gentle with myself. I realize that I'm not bad if I stray, or good if I abstain.
- Give up trying to control anything or anyone outside myself.
- Become increasingly honest and open with at least one other person: my sponsor.
- Accept myself exactly as I am without hiding, distorting, or rejecting any part of myself.
- Forgive myself and others. By blessing those who have harmed me, I find peace instead of resentment.
- To live a joyous, peaceful, fulfilled life, I must engage in a search for my inner strength that I now call God.
- A Power greater than myself is guiding my life whether I recognize it or not.

- Every Step has a principle, and I will be enriched by applying all the Steps in my daily life.
- The promises come true.
- No one ever starves to death between meals.
- To be on amicable terms with my family is a God-given gift.
- Every meeting adds to the recovery.
- I cannot do it alone.
- Half measures avail me nothing.
- Writing is an indispensable method of finding out what's amiss.
- I can live without fear.

— *Anonymous*

The Importance of Being Honest

"If you want to develop self-esteem, you'll have to engage in estimable behavior—behavior worthy of esteem." That's what my sponsor told me throughout the first six months of my program.

Coming to OA 150 pounds (68 kg) overweight and just out of the hospital following two suicide attempts, I was willing to listen to almost anything. But when my sponsor told me this, I was almost at a loss. I had alienated so many people and done so much harm while I was overeating, I doubted I had much to offer. What could I do that was estimable?

Following a lengthy rehabilitation, I was able to return to work for a temporary agency. While on an assignment, an employer asked me to do something which was a clear violation of the law. Since he offered me increased wages, I didn't miss a beat: I gladly accepted the offer. A feeling of misery swept over me. It didn't take much consultation with my Higher Power to understand the cause.

I debated what to do for the rest of the day, and then I explained to my employer that I would be happy to do the work but only in an honest manner. He was caught off guard, as if I'd been the first to turn down his lucrative offer. I was both nervous and excited.

From that day my self-esteem began to grow. My shaky abstinence solidified and has been strong ever since.

We're all given the opportunity to perform estimable acts—sometimes in unexpected ways. I think that means we all have the ability to develop better self-esteem. It's only a decision and an HP away.

— *Winfield, Illinois USA*

A Bouquet For Abstinence

About four months ago, I'd established a working relationship with a loving Higher Power and the food obsession had been removed. Since then I'd been experiencing the "contented abstinence" so often spoken of in OA. One day last week, however, I got into self-pity so intensely that before I knew what hit me, the obsession was back!

I was at work and not feeling well. I'd planned to go home early to try and get some rest, when all of a sudden the idea hit me: "I'll stop by the nearest store on the way home, get all of my favorite binge foods (yes, all of them!) Pile them in front of the TV, and eat—just like old times!" I was actually planning to go through with it. I was tired of feeling bad and desperately wanting a pick-me-up.

Something deep inside shouted at me to stop and think about what I was doing. Did I actually want to get back into that old behavior? "Yes!" I shouted back to the voice inside. "I'll just go ahead and get it over with—then it won't bother me anymore," I rationalized. How many times had I used that line before?

Before I left work I decided to listen to my inner voice for a minute. What was I feeling? What did I really need? "Hmm," I said to myself, "I'm feeling down because I'm sick, and I'm bored from sitting around all week. What I really want is to have some fun!" My old way of having fun was to binge and watch TV. But that didn't work anymore. What else could I do?

I thought for a while about what I might enjoy doing. I love to read, so I decided to go home and curl up with a good book I'd bought a while back and hadn't yet had the chance to read. That sounded like fun. Then I remembered what I'd heard my sponsor say several times: "If you're getting into negative behavior, choose to do something positive to counteract it. It's impossible to be both negative and positive towards yourself at the same time."

Then it struck me: I'd go buy myself some flowers. I immediately forgot all about the planned binge and started thinking about what kind of flowers I could treat myself to. I decided to get the flowers, then spend the rest of the afternoon reading my book and enjoying them. I really got excited about the idea—just as I once did about food.

I headed for the nearest florist. To my delight they had an arrangement designed for sending to a person who needs cheering up. It was just what I needed, filled with colorful flowers and festooned with rainbow decorations. It cost a little more than I had planned to spend, but I recalled all the times I'd spent twice that much on food. I was worth it.

When the woman behind the counter said to go ahead and pick out a card and sign it, I thought, "Why not?" I found one with balloons on it, wrote myself a little love note, and put it in the envelope. I didn't tell her the flowers were for me. It felt kind of neat. I thought of all the times I'd bought huge quantities of food at the grocery store and the funny looks and comments I'd gotten from the people behind the counter. This sure felt a lot better than that.

I had a wonderful afternoon reading my book and enjoying my flowers. The best part is that it's been a week and those flowers still look pretty. If I'd binged it would have been over in about fifteen minutes, and I would have been miserable. Each time I looked at my flowers this past week, I remembered how good it felt to do something loving for myself. Those flowers saved my precious abstinence.

— *Tallahassee, Florida USA*

Young and Abstinent

I came to my first OA meeting one month after my twentieth birthday. My anorexia and exercise bulimia made me feel much older, but I acted like a two-year-old child. This disease is cunning, baffling, and powerful at any age. OA has helped me learn to act my age and enjoy life to the fullest.

That first meeting was more than two years ago, and I have been abstinent for two years and one month. I have gained about 25 pounds (11 kg) in recovery and have maintained a normal weight for almost two years. I look around my home meeting and the other meetings I usually attend and am sad to see that I am still the youngest face around.

I feel lucky to be where I am, but sad to see so many of my peers still suffering. Through this program of attraction and Twelfth-Step work, I have brought some friends to meetings. Some of them have stayed, and it is a joy to see them in recovery. But many are not willing to work this program. The excuses the disease makes are the same at any age. I pray they will come back in time. I need young newcomers to help me as much as they need to be helped. I am thankful that when they make their way back to OA, I will be here—a young person in recovery. For today, all I can do is work my program to the best of my ability.

Other OA members tell me how lucky I am to have found this program at a young age. I thank my Higher Power for that. If I hadn't found OA when I did, I don't know where I would be today, probably dead or in a hospital. I am thankful to OA for giving me my life back.

One advantage to becoming abstinent at a young age is that one day I hope to say, "I have thirty years of abstinence" or even forty or fifty years! One day at a time, I pray that with my Higher Power's help I can say that.

— *New York, New York USA*

Standouts

I'm grateful for my years of abstinence, which started at my second OA meeting in December 1980. I'm grateful to a small woman who approached me, asked if I had a sponsor, and offered to take my call the next morning at 6 a.m. At age twenty-five, I hardly knew 6 a.m. existed, but I did call, and I kept calling. She helped me realize many things, and the following stand out.

> *Abstinence is an act of surrender, not control.*

- Abstinence, which results in physical recovery, is the most important thing in my life without exception. It comes before my relationship with my Higher Power (which would vanish if I went back to the food), my relationships with my family (which would implode), my job (which I would probably lose), and my religion (which would be meaningless).
- Abstinence—being abstinent and staying abstinent—is the greatest service I can do for OA. If I am in the food, then organizing share-a-thons, taking and making calls to newcomers, or speaking at meetings would be merely self-serving and not genuine service to the Fellowship. It could even be harmful to OA as a whole. Being abstinent today shows people the program works. My sponsor told me if I were to relapse, I would have to give up my OA responsibilities, sit down, shut my mouth, and open my ears. She assured me I would have nothing to share if I were not abstinent; I would be as good as drunk. I could still do service by setting out chairs and cleaning up.
- Abstinence does not have to lead to relapse. Recovery is possible in this program just as it is in other Twelve-Step programs. My first sponsor led me through the first nine Steps, an eighteen-month process for me. She expected me to take action on whatever Step I was working on that day and did not let me proceed until I had convinced both of us that I had worked a Step thoroughly and without reservation. Having taken a thorough

Step One, I've never had to reconsider if I am a compulsive overeater. I never have to wonder if my life would be unmanageable if I returned to the food. Having taken a thorough Step Two, I have never had to wonder if there's a way out, a way back to sanity. Having taken a thorough Step Three 27 years ago, I have never had to take back the solo controls for my life, which never worked anyway. I still believe if I work the Step I'm on today (Steps Ten, Eleven, and Twelve), I will not go back to the food. How could I since each day I turn my will and life over to the care of my Higher Power?

- Abstinence is an act of surrender, not control. Eating right was a new concept for me, and letting go of weight control scared me. But I did let go, and I'm so glad! By working the Twelve Steps and living with a desire to not overeat today, I have maintained my weight loss of 30 pounds (14 kg) and done so (except for two pregnancies) for more than twenty-six years. Since I completed Step Nine twenty-six years ago, sanity has become my way of life—not always easy, but always worth it.

I am grateful for my physical, emotional, and spiritual recovery. I am grateful for the opportunities I have to share this amazing program with others. I am grateful for the Steps and my commitment to work the Step I am on today. I am grateful to my Higher Power, who is always within reach, even when I can't sense it. And I am grateful for my first sponsor, who showed me this simple path of recovery out of the food and onto a new plane of existence.

— *Sandwich, New Hampshire USA*

The Twelve Steps of Overeaters Anonymous

1. We admitted we were powerless over food—that our lives had become unmanageable.

2. Came to believe that a Power greater than ourselves could restore us to sanity.

3. Made a decision to turn our will and our lives over to the care of God *as we understood Him.*

4. Made a searching and fearless moral inventory of ourselves.

5. Admitted to God, to ourselves and to another human being the exact nature of our wrongs.

6. Were entirely ready to have God remove all these defects of character.

7. Humbly asked Him to remove our shortcomings.

8. Made a list of all persons we had harmed, and became willing to make amends to them all.

9. Made direct amends to such people wherever possible, except when to do so would injure them or others.

10. Continued to take personal inventory and when we were wrong, promptly admitted it.

11. Sought through prayer and meditation to improve our conscious contact with God *as we understood Him,* praying only for knowledge of His will for us and the power to carry that out.

12. Having had a spiritual awakening as the result of these Steps, we tried to carry this message to compulsive overeaters and to practice these principles in all our affairs.

Permission to use the Twelve Steps of Alcoholics Anonymous for adaptation granted by AA World Services, Inc.

The Twelve Traditions of Overeaters Anonymous

1. Our common welfare should come first; personal recovery depends upon OA unity.

2. For our group purpose there is but one ultimate authority—a loving God as He may express Himself in our group conscience. Our leaders are but trusted servants; they do not govern.

3. The only requirement for OA membership is a desire to stop eating compulsively.

4. Each group should be autonomous except in matters affecting other groups or OA as a whole.

5. Each group has but one primary purpose—to carry its message to the compulsive overeater who still suffers.

6. An OA group ought never endorse, finance or lend the OA name to any related facility or outside enterprise, lest problems of money, property and prestige divert us from our primary purpose.

7. Every OA group ought to be fully self-supporting, declining outside contributions.

8. Overeaters Anonymous should remain forever non-professional, but our service centers may employ special workers.

9. OA, as such, ought never be organized; but we may create service boards or committees directly responsible to those they serve.

10. Overeaters Anonymous has no opinion on outside issues; hence, the OA name ought never be drawn into public controversy.

11. Our public relations policy is based on attraction rather than promotion; we need always maintain personal anonymity at the level of press, radio, films, television and other public media of communication.

12. Anonymity is the spiritual foundation of all these Traditions, ever reminding us to place principles before personalities.

Permission to use the Twelve Traditions of Alcoholics Anonymous for adaptation granted by AA World Services, Inc.

For more information on Overeaters Anonymous,
write to the World Service Office, P.O. Box 44727,
Rio Rancho, NM 87174-4727
or email us at info@oa.org.
Find us on the internet at oa.org.